spike

THE VIRUS *vs* THE PEOPLE
THE INSIDE STORY

Spike – The Virus vs The People: The Inside Story

This paperback edition (with a new Epilogue)
published in March 2022; first editon published in February 2021
by Profile Books Ltd
29 Cloth Fair, Barbican,
London EC1A 7JQ

www.profilebooks.com

Copyright © Jeremy Farrar & Anjana Ahuja

1 3 5 7 9 10 8 6 4 2

The moral right of the authors have been asserted.

All rights reserved. Without limiting the rights under copyright reserved
above, no part of this publication may be reproduced, stored or
introduced into a retrieval system, or transmitted, in any form or by any
means (electronic, mechanical, photocopying, recording or otherwise),
without the prior written permission of both the copyright owner and the
publisher of this book.

A CIP catalogue record for this book is available from the British Library.

ISBN 978-1788169233
eISBN 978-1782839101

Printed and bound in Great Britain by
CPI Group (UK) Ltd, Croydon CRO 4YY
on Forest Stewardship Council (mixed sources) certified paper.

spike

THE VIRUS *vs* THE PEOPLE
THE INSIDE STORY

Jeremy Farrar
with **Anjana Ahuja**

P
PROFILE BOOKS

CONTENTS

1

If anything happens to me, this is what you need to know ...

30 DECEMBER 2019

Known cases: 4

I WAS IN AN AIRPORT lounge on New Year's Eve 2019 when my mobile rang. I was heading back to England from Rwanda and the Democratic Republic of Congo, where I had been visiting the Ebola vaccination centres in Rwanda across the politically fraught border region of North Kivu. I'd spent around a week going around the clinics and I'd had the vaccine myself in Prefegitura ya Cyangugu, a village in Rwanda. I was absolutely knackered and looking forward to a couple of days at home in Oxford before heading back to the office.

I was scanning my phone when I saw a report of a mystery pneumonia spotted by doctors at a hospital in China. I sent a short text message to George Gao, head of the Chinese Center for Disease Control and Prevention (China CDC) in Beijing, and an old friend. George is a very likeable character, as well as a respected scientist, a brilliant impressionist and a karaoke enthusiast. My message was short and simple, just asking if he was OK and that he should reach out if he needed anything.

He phoned me back. Very soon, George told me, the world would be hearing about a cluster of cases of a new pneumonia from Wuhan in China. The cases had already been reported to the World Health Organization. It was, essentially, a courtesy call from one scientist to another. I remember him telling me that we wouldn't need to worry because it wasn't severe acute respiratory syndrome (SARS), and that we must keep in touch.

It was a relief to hear him rule out SARS, a deadly disease that features on the world's worry list and for which there is no vaccine or cure. It first appeared in 2002 – and one of its victims, Carlo Urbani, was a good friend of mine. He died while investigating an outbreak in Hanoi, Vietnam. He was just 46 and had a young family.

Carlo's work helped to identify SARS as a new coronavirus. Most importantly, he spotted that cases of severe pneumonia were being passed on from patients to health workers, who were falling sick and dying. Carlo organised the hospital's closure, alerted the world and, essentially, saved Vietnam. His legacy is honoured, if that is the right word, in the naming of the Urbani strain of the virus. This was the dominant strain that spread across South East Asia in 2003, before being contained, infecting more than 8,000 people and killing nearly one in ten of them.

Having spent eighteen years running an infectious diseases research facility in Ho Chi Minh City, I was badly shaken by Carlo's death. I know what it is like to deal with the science and politics of a new disease. I helped to alert the world to a potentially serious outbreak of H5N1 bird flu in Vietnam in 2004, along with colleagues Tran Tinh Hien, Nguyen Thanh Liem and Peter Horby, then an epidemiologist working for the World Health Organization in Hanoi and now an Oxford University scientist.

Both SARS and H5N1 had a profound psychological impact on me, because of the fear that comes with unknown diseases. They took me back to being a young doctor in London at the start of the HIV epidemic: as medical students and junior doctors we rarely stopped to question the power of medicine, believing unerringly that we could treat people and cure them. But when HIV came along in the early 1980s we could do nothing. Young people would come in to die. The West had not seen deaths from untreatable infectious diseases for many years.

When SARS came, it was the same. You don't know what you're dealing with, you're frightened, friends are dying and it's spreading around the world. Six months later, SARS was finished because it did not transmit readily between people: also, people were most infectious when they were symptomatic. There was little or no asymptomatic transmission, meaning that isolating people with symptoms brought a chain of transmission to an end. Despite lasting only six months, and causing 'only' 774 deaths, the epidemic was estimated to have cost around US $40 billion.

The next year, bird flu struck Vietnam. It never got beyond about 100 cases but it killed roughly 60 per cent of people who caught it. We got lucky because, again, the disease fizzled out. These episodes, along with the emergence and reemergence of other diseases over the last twenty years such as the deadly bat-borne Nipah and Middle East respiratory viruses, and the mosquito-borne Zika virus, were the warnings for what would inevitably come.

✳ ✳ ✳

When I went back to work on Friday 3 January 2020, I emailed two of my most senior colleagues: Eliza Manningham-Buller, the Chair of the Wellcome Trust and former director general of the UK intelligence agency MI5, and Mike Ferguson, her deputy. I would not normally trouble them about a small, distant outbreak – but this one in China felt different. If it turned out to be different, the Wellcome Trust, where I have been director for eight years, would be called upon for its expertise and money. The charity has long worked in the field of infectious diseases, with researchers all over the world; it played a key role in the research response to the Ebola outbreaks of 2014 and 2018, including funding vaccine research and clinical trials.

Prefaced with the line 'Just for info in confidence', I told Eliza and Mike about my phone conversation with George Gao and included a link to a news item on the BBC website about the mystery viral pneumonia from Wuhan. Just before signing off, I speculated that China CDC would make an announcement within 48 hours. I assumed that's what George had meant by his phone call. I reassured Eliza and Mike that 'it is not SARS, although probably a known "relative". Nothing for Wellcome to do at the moment.'

I turned out to be wrong. The cases of unexplained and untreatable pneumonia in Wuhan kept growing, matched later by reports of crowded hospital wards and overflowing mortuaries. Social media and online chat rooms in China hummed with rumours of a strange new illness spreading in Wuhan, including among hospital workers; reports began filtering in of police crackdowns on those trying to get information out over the heavily monitored internet.

By the second week of January, I was beginning to realise the scale of what was happening. I was also getting the uncomfortable feeling that some of the information needed by scientists all around the world to detect and fight this new disease was not being disclosed as fast as it could be. I did not know it then, but a fraught few weeks lay ahead.

In those weeks, I became exhausted and scared. I felt as if I was living a different person's life. During that period, I would do things I had never done before: acquire a burner phone, hold clandestine meetings, keep difficult secrets. I would have surreal conversations with my wife, Christiane, who persuaded me we should let the people closest to us know what was going on. I phoned my brother and best friend to give them my temporary number. In hushed conversations, I sketched out the possibility of a looming global health crisis that had the potential to be read as bioterrorism.

'If anything happens to me in the next few weeks,' I told them nervously, 'this is what you need to know.'

✳ ✳ ✳

The process of reporting a new disease to the wider world is quite informal and not at all glamorous. It often starts with a brief notice on ProMED-mail, an online repository collating short descriptions of outbreaks of animal and human diseases in different countries, as well as other news snippets relating to diseases, such as grant announcements. That is where I had picked up the information on the Wuhan cases that George Gao and I spoke about. The descriptions of outbreaks are clipped from official sources, such as health authorities, but also from social media and local newspapers. Every outbreak that becomes a global headline begins as a local rumour.

ProMED stands for 'Program for Monitoring Emerging Diseases' and is run by the International Society for Infectious Diseases, which boasts more than 80,000 members in 201 countries. It is not sustained by any government or the World Health Organization but by volunteers operating a non-profit initiative on a shoestring budget. It is also far more respected – and critical to global health – than the informal setup would imply. I first became aware of ProMED in 1999, while investigating a mysterious brain infection striking down pig farmers in Malaysia. That turned out to be the first known outbreak of Nipah virus, regarded ever since as one of the world's deadliest disease threats.

The ProMED alert that had caught my eye was dated 30 December 2019, next to a line reading simply: 'Undiagnosed pneumonia – China (HU):RFI'. 'HU' refers to Hubei, the central province in which the city of Wuhan is located: 'RFI' signals a request for further information. The first signs of SARS were cases of undiagnosed pneumonia.

❋ ❋ ❋

Nobody knew it then but that single line marked the debut of a new disease, one that would come to be called Covid-19 and cause the biggest upheaval to the global order since the Second World War. The line clicks through to an imperfect machine translation of a story relating to 'an urgent notice on treatment of pneumonia of unknown cause' originally posted that evening by the Medical Administration of Wuhan Municipal Health Committee, concerning four patients with an unknown form of pneumonia.

A report appended underneath that urgent notice adds worrying detail gleaned on 31 December: 27 people were in various hospitals in Wuhan with viral pneumonia or pulmonary (lung) infection. Two were recovering but seven were critical. Flu and bacterial diseases had been ruled out – but not SARS. Citizens were being urged not to panic.

All the patients apparently had links to the Wuhan South China Seafood Wholesale Market (also known as the Huanan Seafood Market). That market link would have worried scientists like me: crowded and cramped 'wet markets', named for the melting ice that keeps meat and seafood fresh, often sell wild and domestic animals alongside meat and fish. The messy overlap provides contact between species, a common feature in the emergence of new diseases because it opens avenues for microbial traffic. That exchange can be between different animal species and between animal species and humans. The report added: 'At present, related virus typing, isolation treatment, public opinion control, and terminal disinfection are underway.'

Public opinion control. Underneath the news reports, a ProMED moderator made an astute observation. Having been involved in publishing early information about SARS, the anonymous moderator wrote, 'the type of social media activity that is now surrounding this event is very reminiscent of the original "rumors" that accompanied the [SARS] outbreak.' Weibo, the Chinese social media channel, was also buzzing with speculation.

The moderator turned out to be Marjorie Pollack, an American epidemiologist who has worked in 50 countries for the US Centers for Disease Control and Prevention. She noted that the bubonic plague, which had cropped up the month before in Inner Mongolia, was sometimes accompanied by unusual pneumonia but assumed this had been already ruled out in Wuhan (plague is caused by *yersinia pestis*, a bacterium, while the Wuhan pneumonia bore the hallmarks of a viral infection). She appealed for more information, and for the results of any tests.

On 31 December, the WHO requested information from China on the Wuhan cluster of atypical pneumonias.

❋ ❋ ❋

On 3 January 2020, ProMED posted an update pulled from the *South China Morning Post*. The unexplained disease was spreading: 44 patients in Wuhan, up from 27; 11 seriously ill with breathing difficulties and lesions, or scarring, on both lungs. There was another unwelcome development: five people had shown up in Hong Kong with unexplained fever after visiting Wuhan. Yet the Chinese authorities had not yet found – or not yet chosen to disclose – the cause.

By 5 January 2020, the WHO, guided by the official information it was receiving from Wuhan, was reporting that there was no significant evidence of human-to-human transmission. Contact tracing was underway to find those linked to the Wuhan patients, many of whom had been stallholders at the seafood market. The persistent market link, the WHO reported, 'could indicate an exposure link to animals'.

That tight case definition resulted in an Escher's loop of misguided circular reasoning: testing only those people with a link to the market created the illusion that the market was the source of disease, because everyone testing positive had been there. In reality, the net should have been cast wider – and the continually growing casualties should have immediately prompted suspicions of human-to-human transmission rather than infections from a single source, such as a contaminated animal carcass.

The WHO also reported that no healthcare workers seemed to have come down with symptoms: illnesses among nurses and doctors act like a canary in the coalmine for new contagious diseases, because infection takes place before nurses, ambulance drivers and other healthcare staff know what they are dealing with.

But, to any outside observer familiar with China as a scientific superpower, second only to the US in research spending, the ignorance was peculiar. Why did nobody seem to know what Wuhan medics were dealing with? The authorities kept insisting that SARS, influenza and bacterial causes had been ruled out – and yet had not pronounced on what could be ruled in. It was baffling: samples would have been sent from those first patients to laboratories for urgent testing and analysis. There was even a top-level biosafety laboratory in Wuhan, a coincidence that would later fuel theories about the virus's origins. Why had that information, potentially crucial to global public health, not yet been released?

ProMED reported: 'The Chinese Center for Disease Control and Prevention is expected to make an announcement of its findings in the coming days, a person familiar with the matter said. The CDC couldn't be reached for comment late Tuesday [7 January 2020].' The report went on to remind readers that China had covered up SARS when it emerged in 2002, reporting it to the WHO only after it began spreading across and beyond southern China.

Just a week into the new year, the unknown disease was no longer wreaking havoc just in Wuhan, a city of 11 million people and a major travel hub in central China. Authorities in neighbouring Hong Kong and Singapore, having already experienced the unwanted gift of SARS nearly two decades earlier, were now monitoring their borders for passengers with fever. A lot of people were becoming anxious – and for good reason. A week is an unsettlingly long time in the world of infectious diseases.

By Friday 10 January it was clear that the Chinese authorities knew more than they were letting on. Colleagues at the World Health Organization discovered that two scientific papers about this new viral pneumonia were in the pipeline at *Nature* and the *New England Journal of Medicine*, two prestigious journals. Maria Van Kerkhove, an epidemiologist in the WHO's Health Emergencies Programme, alerted me.

It was time to send out a signal. I tweeted:

If rumours of publications on the Wuhan Pneumonia situation are being prepared and submitted to @nature @NEJM are true & that critical health information is not being shared immediately with @WHO – something is very wrong

Within minutes, the tweets attracted a private message on Twitter and a phone call from the other side of the world. Something was, indeed, very wrong.

※ ※ ※

Scientists track how viruses relate to each other by drawing family trees, in much the same way that people can trace their own origins back by following the trail of births, deaths and marriages. Instead of surnames and family records, viruses reveal their origins in their genetic sequences. Genetic overlap pinpoints the similarities between different viruses, signposting when they potentially share a common ancestor. Likenesses between human viruses and animal ones can also narrow down which animal might have transferred a virus across the species barrier to us.

Scientists can then construct a 'phylogenetic tree' that accords the newbie pathogen its rightful place in the viral hierarchy by establishing how closely related it is to other known viruses. This helps virologists to decide whether an emerging virus is a variation on a known virus or a fresh addition to a particular family of viruses. A tree for a virus can be drawn in different ways but often looks like a collection of fork prongs (or tines).

At the tip of each tine lies the name of a virus designed to showcase something of its origins. The pandemic virus that causes Covid-19 is now called SARS-CoV-2: severe acute respiratory syndrome coronavirus-2. The original

SARS virus to which it bears significant genetic resemblance used to be called SARS-CoV and has now been renamed SARS-CoV-1.

Eddie Holmes is a British-born virologist and professor at the University of Sydney who does exactly this sort of viral detective work. He is, in my book, the outstanding evolutionary biologist of his generation, with an extraordinary brain when it comes to pattern recognition.

Eddie belongs to a research consortium which includes the Shanghai Public Health Clinical Center and School of Public Health at Fudan University, Shanghai, where he holds an honorary professorship. Since 2012, Eddie has worked closely with Professor Yong-Zhen Zhang, a professor at Fudan University, on finding and identifying new animal viruses, and Wuhan is a familiar locale in their virus-hunting network.

'We have this little routine,' Eddie says of his work with Zhang trying to document the diversity and evolution of animal viruses. 'His team collect samples – they can be spiders or fish or anything – and then I go over there once or twice a year and help analyse the data.'

They don't normally study samples from humans but genomic sequencing, the method used to place viruses in their family trees, can also be used as a diagnostic, to help identify mystery viruses found in hospital patients. Over the past eight years, Eddie and Zhang, more used to collecting virus samples from cave-dwelling bats than from city dwellers, have built up contacts with Wuhan doctors. As Eddie says, rather honestly: 'The animal stuff is great but everyone wants to find a new human virus. It was obvious that Zhang was going to be one of the first people to get hold of samples.'

On 3 January 2020, Zhang struck viral gold: a sample taken from a pneumonia patient hospitalised in Wuhan on 26

December 2019 arrived at his lab packed in dry ice in a metal box. By 2am on 5 January, after a 40-hour shift in the lab, Zhang and colleagues had worked out its genetic sequence. It was a coronavirus that looked suspiciously like SARS-CoV-1, the virus responsible for the 2002/3 outbreak. Coronaviruses are named for their similarity in appearance to a crown: under powerful microscopes, the virus particles look like tiny spheres covered in small spiky protrusions. Those spikes help the virus get into cells to infect people; most vaccines target the spikes to disrupt the process.

Eddie still remembers the phone call (Sydney is three hours ahead of Shanghai): 'We agreed that he should tell the Ministry of Health in China immediately. Zhang did it the same day.

'Zhang told them it was clearly very closely related to the first SARS virus and that it was very likely to be respiratory because of its relatedness. He also told the ministry that people should take precautions.'

That phrase – 'people should take precautions' – was a direct warning that this new virus, like its dangerous predecessor, might be able to spread from one person to another. Eddie says this should have been interpreted back then as a warning of human-to-human transmission. In the end, China did not confirm this publicly until 20 January, more than two weeks later.

While Zhang informed Beijing, some of the sequence was deposited on 5 January 2020 on GenBank, an online collection of publicly available gene sequences run by the National Institutes of Health in the US. But it takes a while for those deposited sequences to be checked, edited and put through the system in a way that others can use. There was an imperative to post the entire sequence more publicly. Anyone, anywhere, could then use that published information to develop a diagnostic test. The world would, at a stroke, have eyes on the virus.

There was, though, a major hitch: Zhang was told in no uncertain terms not to publish anything. The gagging order, Eddie understood, came from Beijing. The warnings to stay silent were real: medics had already been disciplined by the Chinese Communist Party (CCP) for discussing hospital cases online. One of the earliest whistleblowers, ophthalmologist Dr Li Wenliang, became a potent symbol of China's mismanagement of the emerging crisis: he was admonished for warning hospital colleagues of a dangerous new infection, became infected and died aged just 33. The Chinese government later apologised to his family, including his pregnant wife.

Eddie and Zhang hit on a loophole to get round the gagging order: the government ban on publishing information about the outbreak did not preclude them from writing and submitting a scientific paper. Holmes contacted the journal *Nature*; one of its editors, Clare Thomas, urged them to submit something as soon as possible. By 7 January 2020, Zhang's paper, with Eddie as one of the co-authors, reached *Nature*'s offices in London.

Things began moving quickly and chaotically. On 8 January, rumours began circulating that the new virus was a coronavirus, putting it in the same family as SARS. A day later, the Chinese authorities confirmed the fact. But, otherwise, and especially on the genome sequence of the virus, they were silent. Not only had Zhang contacted China's Ministry of Health with details of the new virus but Eddie was sure that, in doing so, Zhang had merely confirmed information that Beijing already knew. Eddie had screenshots of messages on WeChat, a social media platform in China, suggesting two private companies had already sequenced the virus in December 2019.

Eddie, disturbed at what was looking increasingly like a decision by China to hold back information on a new disease, saw my tweet about the two scientific papers about to come out. His name was on one of them. He rang me to tell me that he'd been trying to get the sequence released, with no luck.

After that call from Eddie, I realised that he and I were probably the only two people in the world outside China who knew there was this sequence in existence and what it was, with all the potential consequences. The information was stacking up: here was a mysterious new pneumonia and, with the sequence, we knew it was caused by a novel coronavirus closely related to SARS. Those are two big red flags.

But the really critical information, the kind that stops you sleeping at night, was still to come.

✱ ✱ ✱

The news of a novel coronavirus outbreak in China at the start of 2020 chilled the blood of scientists, including me, who witnessed the appearance of severe acute respiratory syndrome (SARS) nearly two decades before. That disease, also associated with a fatal pneumonia, first emerged in the Guangdong province of southern China in 2002. It spread largely unchecked in southern China and then crossed borders. By August 2003, it had infected more than 8,000 people in 37 countries and killed 774. That was the virus that killed my friend Carlo in Vietnam.

Like so many of the viruses that feature in epidemiologists' anxiety dreams, SARS-CoV-1 is found naturally in bats – and the animals themselves seem untroubled by viruses that are so virulent in other species. The 2002/3 outbreak is thought to have been triggered by that virus passing from bats to humans via an intermediate species, with civet cats a probable culprit. These long-bodied, short-legged animals, closer in appearance to a mongoose than to a cat, are commonly sold for food and have been found to harbour viruses closely resembling SARS-CoV-1.

SARS is a painful memory in the collective Chinese consciousness – and in the annals of global public health – because the government spent the early months of the epidemic covering it up. In fact, the parallels between that original SARS outbreak, caused by the virus SARS-CoV-1, and the Covid-19 pandemic, caused by the closely related virus SARS-CoV-2, go beyond virus names. Both are likely to have started in November and, while reported up the chain of public health command, failed to properly attract the attention of Beijing until January.

It is an auspicious time of arrival for any malevolent microbe, given the proximity of the Chinese New Year. The week-long holiday is the backdrop to the world's largest annual migration, as around 450 million people criss-cross the country to visit friends and relatives. That mass movement is the perfect spreading opportunity for a virus. The anticipation of a major public holiday is a distraction for otherwise diligent health officials on the lookout for new diseases.

The top-down, hierarchical way in which the Chinese Communist Party runs the country, with a compulsion to control the message, also seems set up to frustrate early disclosure. With the original SARS, three days were reportedly lost due to the lack of suitably senior staff to open a document about the new illness marked 'Top Secret'. When health alerts eventually came, they were sent out during the Chinese New Year, when many hospital staff were absent. It was February 2003 before the World Health Organization was officially notified, by which time more than 300 people had fallen ill. Insistence in Beijing that the SARS outbreak was being contained was followed by an effective news blackout in the run-up to the National Party Congress in March 2003.

In April 2003, a surgeon in Beijing finally blew the whistle, claiming many cases in the capital had been covered up. The authorities in Beijing were slow to consent to WHO requests to investigate. The epidemic, which seeded large, deadly outbreaks in Hong Kong, Taiwan and Canada, was contained by August 2003 but the inglorious debut of SARS still serves as a benchmark for how not to handle a new disease. It took four months for China to report cases to the WHO, and another month before the coronavirus SARS-CoV-1 was unveiled as the pathogen responsible for the disease.

SARS was the costly catalyst for change in China: the country strengthened its disease surveillance network and put in place an online reporting system accessible by any hospital. It wasn't a half-hearted tweaking of the system but a radical rethink: the China CDC became a slick, profes-sional, science-focused organisation, with fresh buildings, a new infrastructure and highly trained staff capable of gracing any world-class research institution – George Gao among them.

But the lessons from SARS still sting. Speed and openness are essential.

That is why Eddie contacted me. He needed to share the burden of the knowledge he had been building up in that first week in January: that the virus responsible for this mysterious pneumonia in Wuhan had been sequenced as far back as December 2019; that Zhang's consortium had a paper waiting to go; and that China knew the virus had been sequenced but had not yet released the information.

Eddie and I had a series of frantic calls between London and Sydney on the night of Thursday 9 January, which stretched into the early hours of Friday. We hatched a plan that Eddie would go back to his collaborators in China and I would go back to George Gao at China CDC. We would threaten to go public if they refused to disclose the information by Saturday morning GMT.

We decided to tell them, 'If you don't release the sequence in the next 24 hours we will release it the next day.' By 9.18pm London time, and 8.18am in Sydney, Eddie and I had committed to the high-stakes pact to force China's hand.

I felt terrible because I'd never done anything like that before – but issuing an ultimatum felt like the only way. News was filtering out about healthcare workers falling sick. Waiting for the wheels of China's bureaucracy to turn quickly enough to make a formal declaration just before Chinese New Year, which lay two weeks away, was too dangerous. It would have taken days and, frankly, we didn't have days. Once it was clear this was a SARS-related coronavirus spread by the respiratory route and that healthcare workers were succumbing, it was clear that things were going to deteriorate quickly.

The world had to have access to that sequence because the world needed to be able to diagnose it. It was going to appear in Beijing, in Hong Kong and Singapore in the hours or days that followed. It was going to spread everywhere.

Eddie remembers the pressure-cooker atmosphere of those days too. Zhang deserved public credit for leading the consortium's sequencing breakthrough – but Eddie also knew his colleague would also be at the sharp end of Beijing's displeasure for shattering the government's code of silence.

'My big concern was not getting Zhang in trouble,' Eddie says now. 'I called him and said, "There's a lot of pressure to release the sequence. I think we have to do it". Zhang was on a plane going from Shanghai to Beijing, on the runway literally waiting to take off.'

Zhang asked his collaborator for a moment to think. It didn't take long. Perhaps Zhang had already decided the world had waited long enough. Before the plane took to the skies, Zhang rang Eddie back with a simple message: 'OK, let's release it.' Eddie phoned me immediately.

By the time Zhang's plane touched down just over two hours later, the information was out.

❊ ❊ ❊

The drama that preceded publication was followed by first comedy and then tragedy.

Comedy, because almost as soon as Eddie had promised to Zhang he would release the sequence, he realised he didn't have it. Eddie had no need of the sequence itself in order to carry out his virological analysis for the *Nature* paper; his contribution just entailed sending suggestions of further work to colleagues in China. A colleague of Zhang's in Shanghai quickly emailed the sequence over.

Without a moment to lose, Eddie rang Andrew Rambaut, an evolutionary biologist at the University of Edinburgh and a trusted contact. The clock was approaching midnight for Andrew but, as Eddie knew, his friend always worked late into the night. Andrew runs an open-source website, virological.org, collating information, including genome sequences, on viruses that might be of interest to other scientists – and agreed during the phone call from Eddie to publish the sequence.

Andrew had no qualms about being an accomplice to the release: 'I've known Eddie for years,' Andrew says. 'I trusted that he and Zhang knew it was the right thing to do. Once it had been quality controlled and we were sure it was the right genome, there was no justification for delay.'

Eddie and Andrew set about compiling all the information that would go public. They wrote a little blurb about what the sequence was, who it came from (Zhang's consortium) and who to ask permission from if anyone wanted to use the data. That blurb went back and forth a few times between Sydney and Edinburgh to make sure it had all the correct information. Andrew immediately uploaded it to virological.org and Eddie posted news of the data release on Twitter.

Eddie is rightly proud of how quickly things happened: 'I've timed it: I had that sequence in my possession for 52 minutes before it was published.' Speed matters perhaps more than anything else in disease outbreaks.

But Eddie had also been so consumed with the cloak-and-dagger intrigue of publishing the sequence that it dawned on him he hadn't stopped to check it before pressing 'upload'. 'It could have been any old shit,' he smiles now, wincing at the memory. 'After I'd posted it, I thought I'd better check it was actually a coronavirus. Luckily it was!'

It was done. At 1.05am GMT on Saturday 11 January 2020, under a week after the virus was sequenced by his colleagues in China, a post entitled simply 'Novel 2019 coronavirus genome' appeared on virological.org, under Eddie's name. A short note underneath explained he was acting on behalf of a consortium led by Professor Yong-Zhen Zhang of Fudan University. The consortium included hospitals and health authorities in Wuhan, plus the Chinese CDC and Sydney University.

I had been on high alert for this moment, and immediately praised the release on Twitter:

Potentially really important moment in global public health must be celebrated, everyone involved in Wuhan, in China & beyond acknowledged, thanked & get all the credit. Sharing of data good for public health, great for those who did the work. Just needs those incentives & trust.'

I wanted to send out the message that fast data-sharing in a global public health emergency is absolutely the right way to go. It opened the floodgates in the way we hoped it would: other researchers jumped on the newly released data and immediately started analysing it. Unsurprisingly, Andrew was one of the first: he concluded there was 89 per cent overlap with a coronavirus found in bats.

The publication, in defiance of the gagging order, seemed to wake China up. Later, on 11 January, China CDC sent the genetic sequence privately to the WHO; the agency responded by saying it hoped China would make the sequence public. This China did, on Sunday 12 January, confirming the sequence that Eddie and Zhang had posted.

As time has passed, Eddie has come to believe the silence from the Chinese government and CDC in the earliest days of January 2020 was down to panic management, control of the message, and, remarkably, the prestige of publishing first. As Eddie puts it: 'They [the Chinese government] didn't want panic, because the word SARS is toxic to them. They wanted to control the message, because that's what China does, and they wanted the big paper themselves. So much of science is about ego, for me as well. Who doesn't want the first paper?'

That the information wasn't shared earlier, Eddie thinks, may also have been down to a miscalculation: that this new virus was sufficiently like the original SARS virus that it would only transmit when people had symptoms. Eddie says: 'I think in early January 2020 people in China thought it would just cause an outbreak in Wuhan. It might get a bit further, but it won't spread that far and they'll control it. I honestly think that's what they thought would happen.'

That delay would turn out to be a misjudgement for both China and the world. Asymptomatic and pre-symptomatic transmission allowed the virus to spread widely: at the beginning of an epidemic, people cannot contain what they cannot see.

If that January weekend opened with a mixture of drama and comedy, it ended on a note of tragedy. On Saturday 11 January came the first reported death from the new corona-virus, a 61-year-old man who regularly visited the seafood market. The day after, Zhang's laboratory at Fudan University in Shanghai was shut down temporarily by the authorities for 'rectification'. It was the price that Zhang, who had set up his own lab partly to cut loose of CDC shackles, would pay for defying the Chinese government.

✴ ✴ ✴

On the day that Zhang's laboratory was shuttered, the WHO released a news update stating it was 'highly suggestive' that the outbreak was related to exposure at the seafood market. The statement noted that no cases had been seen outside Wuhan, downplaying fears that it might be contagious: 'there is no infection among healthcare workers, and no clear evidence of human-to-human transmission'.

By the time this statement was posted, several people inside China must have known this to either be untrue or contrary to emerging evidence. The intelligence came via an email from someone I had worked with before, a researcher at Erasmus University in the Netherlands.

From: T. Kuiken
Date: Saturday, 18 January 2020 at 16:08
To: Jeremy Farrar
Subject: Wuhan coronavirus

Dear Jeremy,
Sorry to bother you on the weekend, but I have a dilemma about not disclosing info about the Wuhan coronavirus that I think should be made public. Do you mind to phone me about this at your earliest convenience at +31 ...

Best wishes, Thijs.

Thijs Kuiken, a veterinary pathologist by training who advises the Dutch government on the threat posed by zoonotic diseases (diseases that are transmitted between species, usually from animals to humans), is one of the unsung scientific heroes of the pandemic. He was sent a research paper on 16 January 2020 by the *Lancet* medical journal, to review for publication. This was one of the standout moments in the whole epidemic, the reddest in a constellation of red flags.

The *Lancet* paper set out how, in early January, a team led by scientists at the University of Hong Kong studied a family of six from Shenzhen, a southeastern city in China, who had travelled to Wuhan over the New Year to stay with relatives. None of them had gone to the seafood market, though two had visited a Wuhan hospital. Five caught the novel coronavirus. On their return to Shenzhen, another family member who had not travelled to Wuhan fell ill.

Here was the critical information that suggested the virus could jump from one person to another, and that it was spreading outside Wuhan. The paper concluded: 'Our findings are consistent with person-to-person transmission of this novel coronavirus in hospital and family settings, and the reports of infected travellers in other geographical regions.'

Even more alarmingly, the paper contained two other vital pieces of information about the new disease: one infected family member was excreting virus without showing any clinical symptoms, suggesting the frightening possibility of asymptomatic spread; and some of the other infected relatives had diarrhoea as their chief or only symptom, which did not feature among the signs that medics had been urged to look out for.

Scientists who review research papers – to check before publication for errors, and that the methods, analysis and conclusion seem reasonable – are sent those papers in confidence. Secrecy is a golden rule for most journals during this well-established checking process, known as peer review. Not only is it a courtesy to peers to judge each other's work in confidence but original research is also harder to get published if it is already in the public domain.

The confidentiality requirement put Thijs in a dilemma: his role as reviewer officially precluded him from sharing the findings – but it meant he was sitting on information that was obviously vital to an unfolding health emergency in which every passing day mattered. And it was information that, for whatever reason, China had not yet disclosed to the WHO.

'I was asked to review the paper within 48 hours so I sent in the review the next day, on the Friday morning,' says Thijs. 'Separately, I immediately contacted the *Lancet* to say the information should be made public because it was the first scientific proof that the virus was spreading human to human. They either would not or could not do it. I also strongly recommended to the authors that they should make the findings public. That did not happen either.'

Thijs spent Friday and Saturday morning monitoring emails, Twitter, ProMED and WHO updates to see if the information had trickled through the system and out into public channels, but there was still no word of human-to-human transmission. That prompted Thijs's email to me on 18 January.

I called him straight back and agreed wholeheartedly that the information should be shared as soon as possible in the interests of public health. If there was a novel contagious disease that could spread asymptomatically between people, and a relative of SARS at that, the world needed to know immediately. I emailed and called the *Lancet*'s editor-in-chief, Richard Horton, left him a message, and took our dog Coco for a walk to clear my head. I emailed Thijs when I got back:

Date: Saturday, 18 January 2020 at 18:11
To: T. Kuiken
Subject: Re: Wuhan coronavirus

Thijs

Thinking aloud whilst trying to get through to Richard.

Option A – Do nothing and wait for it to go through the system

Option B – Leave until Monday and speak with Richard then

Option C – release a summary online such as

Aware of a manuscript submitted which shows

H-2-H transmission within a family cluster in a city away from Wuhan.

That people are viral +ve and may be infectious when asymptomatic/very mild symptoms and afebrile.

That transmission may be by more than respiratory ie diarrhoea.

That this is present in cities in China beyond Wuhan.

That there is ongoing transmission.

Viral sequence available.

Releasing this information for public health benefit.

Encourage those with this (investigators and editors) to release immediately and publish at a later date

Thoughts?

I would be happy to do Option C if you felt appropriate and if you think the summary accurate reflection of the important public health message.

To be honest I was angry that Thijs had found himself in this impossible position. With Thij's permission, I rang Maria Van Kerkhove, from the WHO's Health Emergencies Programme, to alert her, without revealing Thijs's identity. Maria, who I trust completely, immediately saw the seriousness of the situation, and asked for the anonymous reviewer to contact her in confidence.

By Saturday evening, Thijs had had enough. He emailed his contact at the *Lancet* to say that if the information had not been made public by the morning of Sunday 19 January, he would inform the WHO.

In his willingness to go rogue, Thijs made a selfless calculation. He could understand why the *Lancet* was unlikely to break cover: it would be damaging for a prestigious journal to rip up its covenant of confidentiality to scientists submitting manuscripts. He also grasped that the scientists were frightened of going public because the Chinese government was threatening to jail anyone revealing sensitive information about the epidemic. Evidence of human-to-human transmission was about as sensitive as it could get. The shutdown of Zhang's lab after releasing the coronavirus sequence against the will of Beijing, and the arrest of those in Wuhan spreading information on social media, was having the desired chilling effect.

The only thing Thijs had to lose was his reputation – and the trust of his colleagues. Yet he was prepared to make that sacrifice, an enormous one for a leading scientist. He reflects now: 'I knew I would be breaking a very strong rule for a scientist [by going public], and that I might not get sent any more manuscripts for review because journals and scientists might not trust me. But it would just be me who was burnt and I thought it was for the public good.

'I had been involved with SARS and I knew that it was only stopped from being a worldwide outbreak because of good public health measures, plus the fact that the virus was just a little bit too slow. I worried that this new coronavirus was going to be a big pandemic because it was spreading so fast out of Wuhan. There were too many cases to be explained just by direct transmission from animals. There was only a small chance of stopping it, and this information was one of the things that could make a difference.'

In one way Thijs handled it perfectly and correctly: he did not send either me or Maria the paper, only a two-page summary and the conclusion (he did initially think of sending the entire paper to the WHO but could not bring himself to do it). Given the sensitivities, Maria concluded the journal should publish as soon as possible; and meanwhile she began quietly incorporating the possibility of asymptomatic human-to-human transmission into WHO discussions on guidance and actions to be taken by countries.

Thijs could so easily have taken the easy option: reviewed the paper, stayed silent and waited for the news to come out on publication, which could have added weeks of delay. The world should be grateful that he did not.

The next day, on 20 January, China confirmed human-to-human transmission. The paper was published online by the *Lancet* on 24 January 2020. So, it was official: the new decade had recorded its first new highly transmissible viral respiratory disease, which could kill some and yet leave others untouched. Carriers could be both asymptomatic and infectious. The world had no natural immunity to this novel virus, and no diagnostic tests, vaccines or treatments.

The virus had all the makings of a nightmare.

❋ ❋ ❋

Eddie has screenshots taken from social media in China about the coronavirus sequence. They suggest the full genome was known by a genomics company in China by 27 December 2019. It was reported to both China CDC and the hospital who provided the patient sample, on 27 and 28 December. Samples appear to have been sent to a second sequencing company, who provided the sequence by 30 December.

That would fit in with Eddie thinking that Zhang was merely confirming what Beijing already knew.

Something has bothered me since: how could George Gao confidently rule out SARS as the cause of the mystery pneumonia cases, as he asserted to me at the beginning of January, without either evidence or a strong suspicion that it was something else? Good scientists like George don't pluck facts from thin air, nor indulge in random guesswork. George has not replied to requests for an interview but he has assured me he did as much as he could to push information into the public domain, including through international journals, as quickly as possible. I believe he did as much as humanly possible within a system.

Frankly, we don't know for sure how long China sat on any of this information in December 2019. All the elements that Eddie mentioned – about China seeking to control the message and avoid panic, and coveting the first scientific paper – are probably relevant, but it was also nearly Chinese New Year and the middle of the flu season. Sifting out a novel pathogen from lab samples will always be challenging: respiratory samples are filled with microbial bystanders, a cocktail of benign viruses, fungi and bacteria that can obscure a rare interloper. I tend to believe in cock-up as much as conspiracy.

There is, however, one message that must cut through: we have got to be quicker and do better when it comes to novel disease outbreaks. Diagnosis is difficult and must improve: having people come in with a respiratory infection that remains undiagnosed is not acceptable anymore. We must be nimble at spotting clusters of illness, such as among family members, and, especially, taking notice when health workers start falling sick. We should be on high alert for unusual symptoms, particularly in critical care; every epidemic of the past two decades has been spotted by critical care clinicians first. The science needs to be shared more speedily, too. Not immediately releasing the sequence is unacceptable. The lag in reporting the human-to-human transmission that had been discovered weeks before it was revealed in the *Lancet*, hindered the early outbreak response.

If each of these elements builds in a delay of half a week, and you've got five different elements, that adds up to a nearly three-week delay. A hierarchical, bureaucratic reporting line system, from a hospital to a provincial arm of the China CDC to the Beijing CDC and back again, doesn't help, especially around Chinese New Year. That could easily build in another two-week delay. That equates to five lost weeks in which spread could have been contained. Even though sectors like online retail and finance live in an age of real-time digital data flows, public health data flows remain stubbornly analogue.

I often wonder whether London, with its nine million people and many hospitals, could have done any better than Wuhan. We could have had one patient in King's College Hospital in south London, two in University College Hospital in central London, one with relatively mild pneumonia and one in intensive care, and two in the Royal Free Hospital, to the north of the city; perhaps another two who'd commuted north out of London to different towns, and another two who had travelled south. Would we have picked up a handful of unusual pneumonias in such a big city in a month, in the middle of flu season? I doubt it. In 2019, the American Thoracic Society noted that, for most pneumonia patients, the microbe causing the infection is never identified.[*]

In most parts of the world, people with a respiratory infection will not undergo a diagnostic test. Others might get a blood culture; in a few places around the world they might get a swab sent off to check for flu or respiratory syncytial virus, another common respiratory virus. If those came back negative, most doctors would shrug their shoulders and say, 'There's something wrong with this patient but I haven't got a clue what it is. Let's start antibiotics and hope for the best.'

Look what happened with the SARS-CoV-2 variant B.1.1.7, which created havoc in the UK at the end of December 2020

---

[*] Pneumonia is an inflammation of the lungs, and specifically the small air sacs, called alveoli, that make up the lungs. The inflammation can be caused by a bacterium, virus or fungus. The infection causes the air sacs to fill with fluid or pus. Symptoms can run from mild to severe and include coughing, fever, chills and trouble breathing. Infants and the over-65s are most vulnerable.

and was the dominant variant of coronavirus around the globe within three months. The UK reported it to the WHO in December, but it first appeared and was sequenced three months previously, in September. Its prevalence only became an issue once genomic surveillance revealed the variant was linked to a surge of infections in Kent in south-east England.

Knowledge must be shared in hours and days, not weeks, and knowledge must lead to action. China may have delayed releasing the information for two or three weeks in December 2019, but the world had all the information it needed by 24 January: a potentially fatal novel respiratory disease that could spread between people without symptoms, with no vaccines or treatments, that had already ravaged a huge, highly connected Chinese city. Early scientific papers from China were spelling out its grim clinical consequences in patients: early symptoms of fever, dry cough, body aches, headaches, progressing to difficulties with breathing, blood clots, pneumonia and, in the worst cases, wider organ failure and death.

Many countries failed to act for many weeks after, or took too long to convert decisions into action. As the virus stirred, much of the world slumbered.

Instead, the new coronavirus kindled a different kind of interest. That is how I came to possess a burner phone.

2

*What do the Chinese know that we don't?**

20 JANUARY 2020

Known cases: 282.
(China: 278; Thailand: 2; South Korea: 1; Japan: 1)
6 deaths in Wuhan.

ON 20 JANUARY 2020, Tedros Adhanom Ghebreyesus, the WHO director general, texted me. He was due in Davos, Switzerland, next day, for the three-day annual gathering of the World Economic Forum but things were moving too quickly for him to leave Geneva. Could I take on some of his commitments, he asked, while I was at Davos? He was anxious for the world's decision-makers to understand the significance of the new transmissible respiratory virus emerging in China.

He had changed his plans because the WHO was due to hold an emergency meeting on 22 and 23 January. The meeting would establish whether the Wuhan outbreak constituted a Public Health Emergency of International Concern (PHEIC).

---

* 'What does the Chinese government know that we don't know?'
  Stéphane Bancel, CEO Moderna

A PHEIC is defined, under the International Health Regulations that frame the WHO's mandate, as 'an extraordinary event that may constitute a public health risk to other countries through international spread of disease and may require an international coordinated response'. The 'Wuhan coronavirus' (by then named 2019-nCoV, meaning 2019-novel coronavirus) had spread beyond China, with cases detected in South Korea, Japan, Thailand and Singapore. Now the WHO, and Tedros specifically, had to decide whether it posed a threat to the world. Given this was a SARS-like coronavirus known to be passing from person to person, a declaration seemed likely.

The groundwork for these judgement calls is laid by a WHO Emergency Committee, a select band of around 20 unpaid specialists from such diverse fields as virology, infection control, vaccine development and infectious disease epidemiology. One member of the Covid-19 Emergency Committee is Marion Koopmans, a virologist in the Netherlands who would later play a key role in researching the origins of the virus. Members draw on evidence and advice from many others.*

The framework is frustratingly binary: an outbreak either is, or is not, a public health emergency. Both conclusions come with double-edged consequences. A declaration can, usefully, spur countries to act, to prepare for a possible surge in illness, but can also disrupt trade and travel if borders close. Shuttering countries can also stop medical supplies getting to where they are needed.

Shying away from a declaration, on the other hand, might prevent panic but if the globe's top health agency doesn't

---

* One such adviser is Anders Tegnell, the epidemiologist at Sweden's Public Health Agency who advocated against strict lockdowns in his country during most of 2020.

deem an outbreak a global emergency, the world tends to shrug its shoulders.

The last PHEIC came in 2019, when Ebola broke out in the Democratic Republic of Congo (distinct from the biggest recorded Ebola outbreak in West Africa, a 2014 PHEIC). Before that, a declaration was made in 2016 for the Zika virus epidemic in Brazil (the epidemic came to light after doctors noted a rise in the number of babies born with microencephaly, or unusually small heads).

These high-stakes calls can burnish or tarnish a WHO director general's legacy. Margaret Chan, Tedros's predecessor, is believed by many to have taken too long to call a PHEIC in 2014 over Ebola in West Africa. The Ebola PHEIC in 2019 was called at the fourth time of asking: it could, and should, have been called the year before. Tedros accepts that.

A declaration gets things moving, unlocks funds, galvanises leaders – ultimately, it saves lives.

※ ※ ※

The International Health Regulations Emergency Committee teleconference meeting on the novel coronavirus opened in Geneva at midday on 22 January 2020, with a briefing by WHO lawyers. Committee members were reminded of the gravity of their responsibility and urged to act ethically and with a duty of confidentiality. More than four hours later, after hearing about the situation in Wuhan, and China's response, the committee declared itself divided on whether to issue a declaration. By this time, remember, the WHO was privy to information contained in the *Lancet* paper that Thijs Kuiken in the Netherlands was sent in confidence; namely, that there was evidence of human-to-human transmission, including without symptoms.

And then came a dramatic update: word arrived from China that the government was going to take the unprecedented step of locking down its citizens to contain the virus. From 10am on Thursday 23 January 2020, reported China's *People's Daily* newspaper, nobody would be allowed to leave Wuhan apart from under exceptional circumstances. The airport and train stations would be shut; bus, subway, ferry and other transport services, suspended. Citizens would be ordered to stay at home or risk arrest.

Eleven million inhabitants would be trapped inside the city, just two days before the start of Chinese New Year. This would be the biggest recorded quarantine in history. The news sent shockwaves through the WHO and around the world. Tedros had not been informed in advance of China's drastic plan. He asked the Emergency Committee to take this extreme measure into account during their deliberations the following day, when a final decision would be arrived at.

＊＊＊

As the tension was ratcheting up in Geneva, I was co-hosting a lunch in Davos, listening to the head of a global bank telling an audience at the World Economic Forum about his struggle with work-related stress. António Horta-Osório, who ran Lloyds Banking Group until July 2020, revealed how he had sought help from the Priory Clinic, a mental health retreat usually associated with celebrities undergoing rehabilitation for drug and alcohol problems. Most people don't talk frankly about their personal troubles but that's the bizarre thing about Davos: here was a top executive discussing his mental breakdown in front of some of the most powerful people in the world. I can't think of anywhere else that brings people together quite like that – from the worlds of business, money, politics, health, academia, plus global agencies and the world's media.

That is why I have been attending for the past five years. You can reach so many audiences – and, whether we like it or not, capitalists can and mostly do make the world a better place. They certainly have a responsibility to do so. Davos hosted the launches of both GAVI, the Vaccine Alliance, in 2000, and the Coalition for Epidemic Preparedness Innovations (CEPI) in 2017. Both have brought about incredibly positive change: GAVI, by vaccinating more than 800 million children in the poorest countries; CEPI, by financing and developing vaccines for diseases including Nipah fever, Lassa fever, Ebola, MERS and Covid-19 (CEPI gave early financing to the Moderna Covid-19 vaccine). During the past two decades, GAVI has prevented an estimated 14 million deaths.

The lunch at which António spoke was co-hosted by Wellcome and Lloyds and boasted a starry list of guests, including the British model Lily Cole. It was intended to lay the groundwork for the 2021 World Economic Forum, on the theme of mental health, particularly in the workplace.

Instead, rumours of China's mystery pneumonia were swirling everywhere and everyone wanted to know more. When the CNN anchor Fareed Zakaria interviewed the then chief executive of Hong Kong, Carrie Lam, on stage at Davos, he opened not with the pro-democracy protests in the former British colony but with the new disease.

'Let me start by asking you something that's on people's minds right now,' Zakaria said smoothly. 'What can you tell us about the Wuhan virus, or what some people are calling the China virus? How rapidly does it seem to spread? How worried should we be?'

Lam gently reminded Zakaria that it was now being referred to as the novel coronavirus pneumonia and Hong Kong was well prepared: holiday camps were being turned into isolation facilities.

Then she added: 'A couple of hours ago, Hong Kong health authorities have just announced we have the first case of highly suspicious infection in Hong Kong from a passenger from Wuhan ...'

✳ ✳ ✳

For the well-connected delegates at the World Economic Forum, this unknown pneumonia was still happening a long way away. There were no travel restrictions, no social distancing, no masks. The world looked just as it always had.

I appeared at a press conference at Davos on 23 January 2020 with Richard Hatchett, the head of CEPI and a White House adviser during the H1N1 outbreak of 2009; and Stéphane Bancel, the now superstar head of biotech company Moderna. Stéphane was already working with CEPI on other vaccines and only that week had inked an agreement with Richard to start work on a coronavirus vaccine.

The sombre meeting, in a darkened Issue Briefing Room, was briskly chaired by Juliana Chan, a science communicator from Singapore (where I was born). Just before the press conference, Singapore announced its first case of the 'Wuhan virus'. There were one or two Western journalists present but it was mostly Chinese media in attendance.

I was asked to speak first. I was in the spotlight. The truth could not be sugar-coated.

'We are about six weeks into this outbreak and this virus can now clearly spread between humans,' I told the audience, explaining it could be passed on like influenza, through coughing and sneezing. 'It is not SARS. The virus is in a similar family as SARS but this looks different ... and the difference is probably it is easier to pass between human beings. I think we can expect many more cases in China and many more cases in other parts of the world.'

Richard then emphasised how much was unknown, such as how infectious the virus was; the pattern of transmission; the range of symptoms and whether they ran from mild to severe; the exact number of cases; how far it had spread geographically.

It is strange to watch the press conference now, to see how little attention anyone paid to Stéphane. Nobody in the audience asked him a single question. His company had quietly picked up the genetic sequence more than a week earlier, on 13 January 2020, and had already begun prepping to produce a prototype messenger RNA (mRNA) vaccine. This is completely new technology: it injects mRNA, a set of genetic instructions for building a bit of the target virus, so that the body's own cells can make the viral protein in-house, to stimulate an immune response. This technology platform, as we have since learned, has the potential to go much faster than conventional vaccine production.

Stéphane urgently needed cash, he had told Richard a few days before Davos, to turn Moderna's baby steps on this new coronavirus into phase 1 trials. In the end, there were just three days between Stéphane's pitch and Richard's sign-off. The tie-up was being announced at the press conference, along with two other CEPI partnerships (with Inovio, for a DNA vaccine, and the University of Queensland in Australia).

As we sat lined up behind the desk and the microphones, Stéphane could see Richard's and my phones buzzing constantly with new updates from Wuhan. The three of us had been meeting up and pooling information, some of it coming from Wuhan and the rest from contacts in the infectious disease community.

✻ ✻ ✻

In the Q&A session at the press conference, a journalist asked if there was any precedent for China's strict lockdown of Wuhan. Richard pointed out that 'when you don't have treatments and you don't have vaccines, non-pharmaceutical interventions are literally the only thing that you have ... isolation, containment, infection prevention and control, and these social distancing interventions'.

And yes, Richard nodded, there was indeed a precedent: how US cities shielded themselves during the Spanish flu pandemic of 1918. 'We found that cities that introduced multiple interventions early in an epidemic had much better outcomes,' he said.

He was referring to a 2007 study of how 43 US cities responded to the arrival of Spanish flu in 1918: those that closed schools and banned large gatherings for long periods earliest in the pandemic fared best. A comparison of excess deaths per 100,000 of population between September 1918 and February 1919 is instructive: Philadelphia, which had 51 days of closures, but belatedly and with not every measure applied at the same time, saw about 250 excess deaths per 100,000 at the peak; St Louis, which acted early and shut down hard for 143 days, saw 30.

But such measures, Richard added, come with drawbacks: they are hard to sustain and create mass anxiety, making the search for vaccines and treatments even more urgent. That's why CEPI had signed three deals; researchers could start working on vaccines straightaway.

Juliana, the moderator, noted that Chinese New Year lay just two days away, when an estimated 450 million Chinese would normally be on the move. Some had already left. 'In many ways, this outbreak could not be happening at a worse time,' I agreed, unthinkingly clicking a ballpoint pen on and off.

I admitted I'm not a huge fan of travel restrictions because people can get round them by using other routes, though they do usefully signal to the public that the situation is serious. They also buy time to put tried and tested health measures in place: testing, contact tracing and quarantine. It might only be a day, a week or a month, but that is better than nothing. Still, there was a catch: border controls must be put in place early, comprehensively and for a long time, as New Zealand did.

Meanwhile, China's sudden lockdown was adding uncertainty and complexity to the second day of emergency deliberations in Geneva. The WHO Emergency Committee advised Tedros that not much had changed from the day before; they still could not decide whether to declare a global emergency.

It was clear that, at that time, there was more to worry about than the week before. There were mass lockdowns in China; rising concerns in the region and beyond about an entirely new transmissible, untreatable respiratory virus of unknown origin; cases were climbing in China and appearing in other countries. People were beginning to draw parallels with 1918.

For all that, the Emergency Committee still could not make up their minds. Tedros had to come down one way or another. On 23 January 2020, the WHO issued a statement concluding that the pneumonia spreading from Wuhan was not a Public Health Emergency of International Concern.

The committee would meet again in a week, sooner if necessary.

✻ ✻ ✻

Moderna started working on the Wuhan coronavirus in early January as a test run for when a real pandemic hit – never expecting this would be it.

Stéphane recalls: 'Our mindset was, let's do this vaccine to see how quickly we can go, because one day there's going to be a flu pandemic and we'll know what we can do. I was worried it might be a distraction. We already had 20 products [in development] in clinic and it was really busy – there was nobody sitting idle to do the project.' Stéphane made a pact with Anthony Fauci, the director of the National Institute of Allergy and Infectious Diseases (NIAID) in the US: Moderna would make up an experimental vaccine and Tony's labs would do the clinical testing.

Davos changed everything, Stéphane told me later. The three of us – Richard, Stéphane and I – were texting each other and grabbing quick coffees between sessions so we could share the real-time updates coming directly from contacts on the ground in Wuhan, which were ahead of the officially reported figures. We were scribbling back-of-the-envelope calculations of how the new coronavirus was spreading, and sketching out scenarios on paper napkins (I wish I had kept the napkins). We were getting case descriptions of patients' symptoms from ground zero, which was exactly the kind of intel that Stéphane wanted to know; Richard and I were laying out everything we knew about coronaviruses.

During one of our meetings, Stéphane realised how little he knew about Wuhan. He recalls: 'I was a bit slow. I knew it was in China but I didn't know how big it was. So, I get my iPad out during of one of the coffee chats and find it's this big industrial city. And then I look at the flights out of Wuhan and realise they go to all the Asian capitals, all the European capitals, and all the big cities on the West Coast of the US. I remember looking up and saying, "Oh shit, it's everywhere".'

It was while we were in Davos that China locked down Wuhan. Stéphane ran into us the next morning, saying 'Jeez, I don't remember any government shutting down a city of that size – ever. What does the Chinese government know that we don't know?'

That was when he knew Moderna had to get serious about its hastily convened side-project. He was meant to be in Germany the weekend after Davos for a business meeting but woke up in a sweat one night, convinced he had to change plans. Stéphane cancelled, sent his apologies and asked his assistant to book him a one-way ticket to Washington DC.

He arranged back-to-back meetings in DC with: Tony Fauci; John Mascola, head of the Vaccine Research Centre at the National Institutes of Health (NIAID comes under the NIH umbrella); and John's deputy Barney Graham, who would fix up the vaccine trials. He also trudged round an alphabet soup of organisations involved in epidemic response: DARPA, BARDA and the FDA.*

'I have never done a thing like this in my life – gone somewhere not knowing when I'm going to come back,' Stéphane says now. 'But that week, and those days at Davos, really changed my mind from, "This is an outbreak" to "Shit, this is a

---

* DARPA (Defense Advanced Research Projects Agency) is a research and development agency of the US Department of Defense. BARDA (Biomedical Advanced Research and Development Authority) is a US Department of Health and Human Services office responsible for the procurement and development of medical countermeasures, principally against bioterrorism, as well as pandemic influenza and emerging diseases. The FDA (Food and Drug Administration) is a US federal agency responsible for protecting and promoting public health.

pandemic like 1918 and it's going to affect the entire planet for a long time". I have worked in infectious diseases for 25 years and knew every day mattered, because of exponential spread. I knew we had to start running for our lives with the vaccine.'

There followed a heartbreaking struggle during the spring of 2020 to raise money to build manufacturing lines, which saw him touring the world pleading for cash: 'I begged the entire planet: foundations, governments, heads of state. In May I hit my lowest point. I was so depressed and upset because I felt I'd failed the world.'

But on 18 May 2020, within five months of the novel disease coming on to the world's radar, the first promising results landed from the phase 1 clinical trials. The vaccine, code-named mRNA-1273, was safe, well-tolerated and, crucially, producing the right kind of antibodies in participants.

Moderna was about to tout for more investment when a call came through from James Gorman, CEO of Morgan Stanley. It was the lifeline that Stéphane had been hoping for: 'He was like, "I don't want you to waste time, you need to focus on the vaccine. The bank will buy the stock and take the risk to sell it back to investors."'

When the markets closed that day, Gorman made good on his promise to the tune of $1.3 billion. For Moderna, at least, the race to a vaccine was back on.

❋ ❋ ❋

By the last week in January 2020, many of us feared the number of cases in China was the tip of an iceberg, because of mild or asymptomatic cases accumulating unseen beneath the surface, as that early *Lancet* paper had suggested. I was baffled by the WHO's decision not to declare a health emergency, as was Tony Fauci in the US.

At Davos, Richard Hatchett from CEPI began looping me into emails with people in the US who were trying to parse the size of the threat and how to get ahead of it. The group included figures in Homeland Security, healthcare companies, the army and public health; they would each bring one or two other voices into the loop to crowdsource information. It was driven by a fascinating left-field thinker called Carter Mecher, who Richard had met during his time advising the White House. Carter is a doctor and former public health adviser in the US Department of Veteran Affairs. He had also worked on pandemic preparedness under George W. Bush, and his emails brought some of the old team together (they had called themselves the Wolverines, after the fictional Marvel Comics character with superhuman senses). By 22 January, Carter had pulled together a quick comparison of SARS, MERS and the new coronavirus and wrote: 'This is taking off faster than SARS...' Early on, he was advising we assume some asymptomatic transmission.

Carter brought incredible insight into those nascent discussions, translating information from China and pointing out that, as had happened with disasters such as the *Deepwater Horizon* oil spill and the Fukushima nuclear accident, public blogs would be a valuable source of inside information and scattered with the technical detail we needed to make forecasts (among those he recommended was flutrackers. com). By 23 January, Carter had pulled together an Excel spreadsheet with case numbers pulled from ProMED-mail and various blogs, coupled with dates of when people had fallen ill and died. His verdict? '[We are] not going to be able to outrun it.' Back then, he was already mooting TLC, or 'targeted layered containment', the kind of measures that many countries would eventually adopt.

That was the day that Wuhan was locked down. It was also the day that he asked us all a question that would stay with me: 'Two weeks from now, are there things that we wished we could have done to reshape the challenge we will likely face? ... We have a very narrow window to act.'

The aim, Carter said, was to 'shape the battlefield'.

※ ※ ※

After Davos, I was sure this was turning into a global pandemic. I discussed with Patrick Vallance and Chris Whitty, the UK government's chief scientific and medical advisers, how the country should prepare and that we should try to start vaccine clinical trials as soon as possible in case US President Donald Trump refused to share future American-made vaccines. I harboured reservations about the lacklustre reaction in the UK. There was a notable lack of public communication on what was unfolding abroad and intensive care units across the UK were already running at full capacity, which has, unfortunately, become the norm.

At my own organisation, Wellcome, a contingencies team was already contemplating the possibility of home working, travel disruption and school closures. As I wrote in an email sent (apologetically) on Saturday 25 January 2020 to a handful of colleagues:

This cannot be contained in China. and will become a global pandemic over the next few days/weeks of uncertain severity. Since Influenza 1918 things have never turned out quite as bad as they appear early on ... but this is the first time since SARS I have been worried ... I worry they [the UK government] are underestimating the potential impact.

On Monday 27 January, I joined a teleconference that brought together, among others, chief scientific adviser Patrick

Vallance (he organised the meeting); chief medical adviser Chris Whitty; Mark Walport, who then led the government funding body UK Research and Innovation (and my predecessor as Wellcome Trust director); Jonathan Van-Tam and Jenny Harries, England's deputy chief medical officers.

That crucial call listed the first steps the UK needed to take to get on top of vaccines, treatments and diagnostics, such as scouting out experts on coronaviruses, issuing a call to vaccine research groups (we expected Imperial College in London and Oxford University to apply, and both duly did), and asking the national drug regulator to streamline its approval process. One suggestion aired at that conference was for Porton Down, the government's top biohazards laboratory, to work on developing a diagnostic test for asymptomatics, the hidden spreaders who carry the virus without showing symptoms.

But at the time a new and even deeper crisis was brewing. After the genetic sequence of the virus was published, people began noticing something peculiar about its molecular structure. In the last week of January 2020, I saw email chatter from scientists in the US suggesting the virus looked almost engineered to infect human cells. These were credible scientists proposing an incredible, and terrifying, possibility of either an accidental leak from a laboratory or a deliberate release.

That got my mind racing. This was a brand-new virus that seemingly sprang from nowhere. Except that this pathogen had surfaced in Wuhan, a city with a BSL-4 virology lab which is home to an almost unrivalled collection of bat viruses. 'BSL' stands for 'Biosafety Level' and 4 is the highest designation, indicating authorisation to handle the nastiest pathogens known to humankind, such as the Ebola and Marburg viruses.

These kinds of labs are, unsurprisingly, rigorously controlled environments: the air is filtered; the water and waste is treated before it leaves the lab; workers change into hazmat suits and shower before and after stepping inside the containment facility. The BSL-4 at the Wuhan Institute of Virology (WIV) is built above a flood plain to withstand a magnitude-7 earthquake. The security in these labs around the world is remarkable.

It seemed a huge coincidence for a coronavirus to crop up in Wuhan, a city with a superlab. Could the novel coronavirus be anything to do with 'gain of function' (GOF) studies? These are studies in which viruses are deliberately genetically engineered to become more contagious and then used to infect mammals like ferrets, to track how the modified virus spreads. They are carried out in top-grade containment labs like the one in Wuhan. Viruses that infect ferrets can also infect humans, precisely the reason ferrets are a good model for studying human infection in the first place. But GOF studies always carry a tiny risk of something going wrong: the virus leaking out of the lab, or a virus infecting a lab researcher who then goes home and spreads it.

GOF studies polarise opinion among specialists and the public. The studies tend to focus on worrisome flu strains like H5N1, which I tackled in Vietnam, and H1N1, which caused a pandemic in 2009 (it came to be known as swine flu because parts of the virus matched flu viruses that commonly circulate in pigs). Many scientists believe such studies are a necessary evil to prepare against future pandemics and to get ahead on vaccines. Others disagree, instead believing that public health goals are more meaningfully served by improving vaccine production or honing our ability to predict pandemics. I believe, broadly, that GOF research can furnish scientific findings that are ultimately useful. Bans are often unworkable in practice; it is better to be transparent and regulate – and such studies are heavily regulated.

The novel coronavirus might not even be that novel at all. It might have been engineered years ago, put in a freezer, and then taken out more recently by someone who decided to work on it again. And then, maybe, there was ... an accident? Labs can function for decades and often store samples for just as long. In 2014, six old vials of freeze-dried variola virus, which causes smallpox, were uncovered in a lab in Maryland, US; though the samples dated back to the 1950s, they still tested positive for variola DNA. Some viruses and microbes are disturbingly resilient.

It sounded crazy but once you get into a mindset it becomes easy to connect things that are unrelated. You begin to see a pattern that is only there because of your own starting bias. And my starting bias was that it was odd for a spillover event, from animals to humans, to take off in people so immediately and spectacularly – in a city with a biolab. One standout molecular feature of the virus was a region in the genome sequence called a furin cleavage site, which enhances infectivity. This novel virus, spreading like wildfire, seemed almost designed to infect human cells.

To say that all this worried me would be an understatement. US–China politics were in a bad place in January 2020; a trade war that started in 2018 with import tariffs was escalating, with high-profile Chinese companies being put on export blacklists. It was obvious that people would soon begin hunting for a scapegoat for what was rapidly turning into a global health disaster. Trump was seeking to blame the virus on China and was calling it the 'China virus' and 'kung flu'. The security services in the US were on high alert for any hint that would prop up the accusations.

Conspiracy theories that were circulating about the origins of the virus were bound to add fuel to an already raging fire.

The rumours centred on the virus being man-made and then either accidentally leaked from a laboratory or, worse, deliberately released. In effect, one idea that was spreading was that the novel coronavirus might be a bioweapon. I remember sitting in the kitchen with my wife Christiane and saying, 'This could be an engineered virus. It could be a lab accident – or worse.' Saying it out loud felt like a bombshell.

It's sobering to look back on it now but there we were, sitting in our home in leafy Oxford, potentially caught up in one of the most polarised moments in history since the Cold War. And sitting on a suspicion that was terrifying – and explosive, if true. This period was much more frightening and uncertain than discussions around the release of the genome a fortnight earlier. With extremely tense US relations and an unpredictable American president determined to see a biological threat through the distorting lens of nationalism, it didn't feel too melodramatic to wonder if an engineered virus, either accidentally leaked or intentionally released, might be the sort of thing countries could go to war over.

Christiane, who is Austrian, is a very calm, pragmatic and logical person. She's also a professor in tropical diseases at Oxford University and knows her immunology. She told me, correctly, that I couldn't get stuck on this idea that the virus was man-made: 'Jeremy, you have to go through the science, you have to look at far more sequences and you're going to have to bring people together. Oh, and you're not an evolutionary biologist.'

❊ ❊ ❊

The idea that an unnatural, highly contagious pathogen could have been unleashed, either by accident or design, catapulted me into a world that I had barely navigated before. This issue needed urgent attention from scientists – but it was also the territory of the security and intelligence services.

I had overlapped with the security services once before, when I was trying to drum up interest in the record Ebola outbreak in West Africa, which started in 2013. Epidemics are as politically destabilising as wars: they spread chaos along with disease. Back then I had trudged to Whitehall to try to convince the security services that the outbreak mattered, because it was threatening to creep into conflict zones. They really do keep a low profile – I remember being sent to an unmarked office down a nondescript corridor.

There is mutual gain to be had from scientists sharing insights with spooks. Just as Wellcome could offer wisdom on how to tackle disease outbreaks, civil servants offered a valuable perspective on the ethnic and political rivalries in North Kivu, the contested border region between the Democratic Republic of Congo and Rwanda. That knowledge greatly helped my Wellcome colleagues working on the Ebola frontline. Andrew Parker was the head of the UK intelligence service MI5 at that time; he has since moved on, but we also spoke about the coronavirus outbreak in early 2020, when he was visiting Wellcome chair Eliza Manningham-Buller, his predecessor at MI5.

When I told Eliza about the suspicions over the origins of the new coronavirus, she advised that everyone involved in the delicate conversations should raise our guard, security-wise. We should use different phones; avoid putting things in emails; and ditch our normal email addresses and phone contacts.

Use different phones? These are not things that normal people do and I had no idea where to start. I contacted the communications tech manager at Wellcome:

27 Jan 2020, at 11:59:

Special request!

Can I get a second phone today? Separate number, need to have one separate to my existing Wellcome one, I hope just for 3–6 months – can explain when we meet

He found me a blank phone in the Wellcome cupboard and left it charging on my desk while I was in a meeting. I didn't know the term then but I now had a burner phone, which I would use only for this purpose and then get rid of.

When I got home, Christiane insisted I rang people close to us, so they would understand what was going on in case anything happened to me.

First, I dialled my older brother Jules, a designer and landscape architect in Edinburgh. I told him that a few scientists, including me, were beginning to suspect this might be a lab accident because it looked, at first glance, as if the virus might not be a natural thing – and, if that turned out to be the case, it would have massive implications for everyone and everything. I told him the British and American intelligence services were involved.

I don't recall him saying very much. What can anyone say? Jules phoned me back about an hour later, to make sure he'd understood it all correctly. And, of course, to run through the usual things you'd expect anyone in his situation to say. Like, if Christiane or the children needed anything, they should let him know.

I had a much longer conversation with Tim.

* * *

Tim Cook is a consultant and professor in anaesthesia and intensive care medicine at the Royal United Hospitals in

Bath, in south-west England. He is one of my closest friends, ever since we were thrown together 35 years ago during our clinical training at the now-vanished Westminster and Charing Cross Hospital.

I came from University College London; Tim, from Cambridge University. We both loved rugby and cricket and we ended up in the same social group. We also shared an intellectual interest in our chosen profession. As Tim says, you would expect everyone who is studying medicine to be really interested in it, but that is not always so.

Tim has been a sounding board, particularly on matters of intensive care, ever since. He was one of the first people I contacted when I began worrying, as coronavirus crept closer, about how health systems would cope with a surge. In late January, after getting off the phone to Wuhan, I emailed him to tell him the situation was worsening fast and doctors were dying. I wanted him and his colleagues to know what might be coming and I wanted to know if the NHS was prepared (his answer was no).

When I worked in Vietnam, he and his colleague Jerry Nolan, who wrote the go-to textbook on emergency care anaesthesia, used to fly out every couple of years to give lectures and train local doctors. In turn, they were tutored by my local colleagues about less familiar tropical diseases such as dengue and malaria.

When I moved back to the UK, Tim smoothed my passage into an amateur cricket club near Oxford. He and I now meet at least once a year for an annual friendly. The pandemic, incidentally, cost me my chance at the rotating captaincy; I'm a batsman and I had been looking forward to becoming the Joe Root of Steeple Aston during the 2020 season. I love cricket; it's pure escapism on a Sunday afternoon in beautiful surroundings, where you can stop thinking about work for a few hours.

No matter what you do for a living, there are always irritations, tensions and stresses. On the pitch, nobody gives a toss about who you are or what you do. We all need places like that, whether it's playing a sport or being in an orchestra – a box where the rest of the world becomes irrelevant.

When I dialled Tim, he was on call in intensive care. He told me afterwards that he would not have answered had it been my usual number. On-call doctors never turn down mystery numbers in case it's an emergency admission, such as a patient with sepsis (a potentially fatal immune overreaction to an infection).

He could hear the fear in my voice and, in turn, it made him nervous. I told him that there were concerns that the virus might be man-made – and that I was letting him know what was going on in case anything happened to me.

'It was a pretty scary call to get from a mate,' Tim says now, recalling it only lasted two or three minutes. He retreated into a sideroom, with nurses and doctors coming in and out. 'I was lost for words and my head was spinning. Your mind races when you hear something like that. If this is an experimental virus that's fallen out of a lab somehow, or been intentionally released, the implications are absolutely massive. So, I'm immediately thinking, this goes from being an absolutely horrendous epidemic to potentially a global disaster with implications for a war.'

Tim didn't tell anyone, not even his wife, for months. Information like this feels like a burden. The last thing you want to do is weigh down anyone else.

The only other time he can remember being as shocked was three years before, again doing a ward round in intensive care. A paramedic rang him from the back of an ambulance: 'Tim, I've got your dad. He's just had a heart attack and I'm bringing him to your department.'

❋ ❋ ❋

Days after I returned from Davos, Eddie Holmes was on his way home to Sydney from another Swiss ski resort. He had travelled to Grindelwald to attend the 30th Challenge in Virology, an annual conference held by the Swiss Academic Foundation for Education in Infectious Diseases.

His scheduled talk was on the emergence and evolution of infectious diseases, and how RNA viruses move from one species to another. When he got there, he and another delegate, Isabelle Eckerle, a virologist at the University of Geneva, delivered an impromptu session on the new coronavirus that everyone was talking about.

The conference was also a chance to take his family skiing – and to take his mind off the constant worry of what was happening to Zhang in China, after the release of the coronavirus sequence without the approval of the Chinese government.

Eddie was in a hotel in Bern when my email landed on 28 January, requesting a chat about the possibility that the virus might have escaped from a lab, given the presence of a BSL-4 facility in Wuhan. I gave him the number of the burner phone to call.

He was tired from travelling and my message was the last thing he wanted to deal with. Still, he pulled out his laptop and began searching for scientific papers that might offer a comparison between the new respiratory virus and its closest known relatives in the animal kingdom. Among a bunch of preprints on BioRxiv,* he found a spot-the-difference paper

---

* Preprint servers are online repositories of draft manuscripts that have not yet been published in an academic journal. The drafts can be checked and commented on by others before formal submission to a journal. Preprint servers such as medRxiv (pronounced med-archive) have allowed pandemic-related research to be disseminated rapidly in the interests of public health, though the lack of peer review means that poor-quality studies can also slip through.

showing how closely this new human virus, then called 2019-nCoV (short for '2019 novel coronavirus') resembled a bat coronavirus.

Despite scanning the pictures and graphs, he could not easily discern any discrepancies between the bat virus and the human one – at least, none that spooked him. After all, if an animal virus has simply crossed over into humans, then the genetic sequences in the virus samples taken from the two species should, genetically speaking, line up pretty well.

And they did seem to marry up, Eddie recalls: 'The virus in humans seemed to have the same variability as the closest related bat virus. If it had been engineered, you'd expect its evolution to look a bit different. I didn't think much of it, if I'm honest. I was busy travelling and trying to write a scientific paper.'

The indifference soon evaporated. The day after arriving back in Sydney, Eddie opened an email from Kristian Andersen at Scripps Research Institute in California, asking for a Zoom call. Kristian has conducted major international collaborations investigating how deadly pathogens, such as Ebola, Zika and Lassa viruses, emerge, spread and evolve. It was only a matter of time before the Wuhan coronavirus, as it was still being called, fell under his lab's scrutiny.

During the call, Kristian confessed to Eddie that three things bothered him about the new virus. The first was that the receptor binding domain, the bit of the spike protein in the virus that attaches to the host cell to infect it, looked too good to be true – like a perfect 'key' for entering human cells.

The second klaxon was that this 'key' was accompanied by a short genome sequence known as a furin cleavage site, seen in highly contagious flu viruses. 'It kind of gives flu superpowers, by making it more transmissible and more pathogenic', Kristian explains, 'and we had never seen it before in these coronaviruses'. If someone had set out to adapt an animal coronavirus to humans by taking a specific bit of genetic material from somewhere else and inserting it, this was what it might end up looking like.

And then Kristian delivered his denouement: he'd found a scientific paper where exactly this technique had been used to modify the spike protein of the original SARS-CoV-1 virus, the one that had caused the SARS outbreak of 2002/3. At first glance, the paper Kristian had unearthed looked like a how-to manual for building the Wuhan coronavirus in a laboratory. The pair knew of a laboratory where researchers had been experimenting on coronaviruses for years: the Wuhan Institute of Virology, in the city at the heart of the outbreak.

'Fuck, this is bad,' was Eddie's first reaction to Kristian's observations. His second instinct was to call me on the burner phone.

3

*Am I supposed to call the FBI?**

30 JANUARY 2020

Known cases: 7,834
China: 7,736 (plus 12,167 suspected)
98 cases in 18 other countries
170 deaths

I GOT EDDIE'S CALL on the day that the WHO's Emergency Committee met for a second time, on 30 January 2020. By now the disease had reached Europe: Germany's Patient Zero, confirmed on 27 January, was a worker at a Munich car factory infected by a colleague visiting from Shanghai, a spark that led to four generations of infection. The virus was on a relentlessly upward trajectory.

At last, the Emergency Committee was unanimous. On 30 January, after a five-hour teleconference, Tedros, on behalf of the WHO, declared the novel coronavirus 2019 a Public Health Emergency of International Concern. It was

---

* 'How do we even do this? Am i supposed to call the FBI?'
Kristian Andersen, Scripps Research Institute, California

belated acknowledgment of what many of us already feared: everything was going the wrong way, and the epidemic was spinning out of control. But at least the declaration would put countries on notice that they had to act under the International Health Regulations, such as to notify the WHO of cases.

The next day, I contacted Tony Fauci about the rumours over the origins of the virus and asked him to speak with Kristian Andersen at Scripps. We agreed that a bunch of specialists needed to urgently look into it. We needed to know if this virus came from nature or was a product of deliberate nurture, followed by either accidental or intentional release from the BSL-4 lab based at the Wuhan Institute of Virology. Depending on what the experts thought, Tony added, the FBI and MI5 would need to be told.

I remember becoming a little nervous about my own personal safety around this time. I don't really know what I was scared of. But extreme stress is not conducive to thinking rationally or behaving logically. I was exhausted from living in two parallel universes – my day-to-day life at Wellcome in London, and then going back home to Oxford and having these clandestine conversations at night with people on opposite sides of the world. Eddie in Sydney would be working when Kristian in California was asleep, and vice versa. I didn't just feel as if I was working a 24-hour day – I really was. On top of that, we were getting phonecalls through the night from all over the world. Christiane was loosely keeping a diary and recorded 17 calls in one night.

It's hard to come off nocturnal calls about the possibility of a lab leak and go back to bed. I'd never had trouble sleeping before, something that comes from spending a career working as a doctor in critical care and medicine. But the situation with this new virus and the dark question marks over its origins felt emotionally overwhelming. None of us knew what was going to happen but things had already escalated into an international emergency.

On top of that, just a few of us – Eddie, Kristian, Tony and I – were now privy to sensitive information that, if proved to be true, might set off a whole series of events that would be far bigger than any of us. It felt as if a storm was gathering, of forces beyond anything I had experienced and over which none of us had any control.

❋ ❋ ❋

Kristian remembers that anxious time at the end of January 2020. 'I drank about three beers after that early call with Eddie,' he says. My overriding concern was to get to the bottom of the origins of the virus as quickly, calmly and scientifically as possible. The first task was to discreetly gather a panel of top-class scientists to ponder aloud about what we were dealing with. I set up a conference call.

We already had Eddie and Kristian. They had been having conversations in the background with Andrew Rambaut and Bob Garry, an expert on viruses at Tulane University in Louisiana and one of Kristian's regular collaborators. Bob had independently clocked what looked like peculiarities in the virus. Kristian had also sought the opinion of his Scripps colleague Michael Farzan, who had made important discoveries about how SARS-CoV-1 binds to human cells.

Michael confessed he was struggling to figure out how the new coronavirus could have acquired its features in a natural way. My wife Christiane recommended Marion Koopmans and Ronald Fouchier, both at Erasmus University in the Netherlands, plus Christian Drosten, who directs the Institute of Virology at the Charité Hospital in Berlin. Christiane pointed out that a truly international group would scotch any rumbling that this was a conspiratorial Anglo-American stitch-up against China.

The panel made a dream team: all globally respected, opinionated scientists who would challenge each other without fear or favour. Marion serves as a science adviser to the WHO – we work together on the science advisory committee for the WHO R&D Blueprint, which focuses on the research strategy for new diseases – and was a member of the Emergency Committee that declared the public health emergency. Later, she would also form part of the WHO delegation that went into Wuhan to investigate the origins of SARS-CoV-2. Ron is a renowned virologist who is a long-time advocate, and practitioner, of gain of function studies. He would be able to give us an insider's view of how likely this kind of research might be at the heart of the mystery.

There was derision down the phone line.

Eddie recalls: 'The general feeling from the biologists was that they just didn't believe a word of it. They could not countenance the fact it might be a lab escape, for good reason: if someone was engineering a coronavirus, they wouldn't use some random bat virus in their own lab. They'd use a familiar strain that they knew could infect cells.' Marion, who did her PhD on coronaviruses, took this view, as did Ron and Christian Drosten. She says: 'There was just no close genetic backbone in the literature, despite there being hundreds and hundreds of genomes of SARS-like viruses in the databases. If you are going to make something, why wouldn't you use one of those to play with?

This novel coronavirus did, at first sight, seem to be a random bat virus – one not specifically documented before either in nature or in the lab. Its closest relative, RaTG13, a 96 per cent match, had just been sequenced but not yet published; I had got hold of a preliminary analysis. It had come from a horseshoe bat and it seemed reasonable to assume this novel coronavirus had come from a bat too. RaTG13 was a closer fit than the two viruses, ZXC21 and ZC45, that Kristian and Andrew had previously been looking at, which were a 86 to 87 per cent fit.

There was a difference of opinion on whether the molecular features were a cause for alarm: nature is a fearsome conjuror, and strange characteristics, like the furin cleavage site in the genome sequence that was catching everyone's eye, can crop up and then vanish through natural evolution. 'You get insertions like that in viruses all the time,' Marion says. 'It happens in nature.' Kristian cautioned that just because it happened in nature did not rule out unnatural origins, especially as closely related coronaviruses lacked some of the same structural features. Ron, meanwhile, worried that focusing on what seemed like an outlandish question would end up distracting busy researchers.

We needed to solicit further opinions, especially as Eddie and Kristian were still nursing concerns. 'At that point,' confesses Eddie, 'I was about 80 per cent sure this thing had come out of a lab.' Kristian was about 60 to 70 per cent convinced in the same direction. Andrew and Bob were not far behind. I, too, was going to have to be persuaded that things were not as sinister as they seemed.

Patrick Vallance informed the intelligence agencies of the suspicions; Eddie did the same in Australia. Tony Fauci copied in Francis Collins, who heads the US National Institutes of Health (the National Institute of Allergy and Infectious Disease, which Tony heads, is part of the NIH). Tony and Francis understood the extreme sensitivity of what was being suggested, given the anti-China rhetoric coming from both President Trump and US Secretary of State Mike Pompeo. Christiane's advice kept running through my head: 'Stick to the science'.

* * *

The next challenge was to find an appointment for a secure conference call that could bring in extra voices. We settled on Saturday 1 February 2020 at 7pm GMT, which was 2pm for Tony in Washington and 6am Sunday for Eddie in Sydney. Kristian and Eddie asked Andrew Rambaut and Bob Garry to dial in. The others on the call were: Francis Collins; Ron Fouchier, Marion Koopmans, Christian Drosten; Stefan Pohlmann, a virologist at the German Primate Centre in Gottingen; Mike Ferguson, Wellcome's deputy chair and a biochemist; Paul Schreier, also from Wellcome; and Patrick Vallance.

Ron, Marion and Christian again argued there was no need to invoke an unseen hand to cook up this particular coronavirus. The ingredients were probably out there in the wild, given that animal viruses are known to cross over into humans all the time or cross over into other species and then into people, where again they mostly hit a wall. The new virus was more convincingly explained, scientifically, as a natural spillover than a laboratory event. The call lasted around an hour; I remember Francis having to step out of his granddaughter's swimming gala because he couldn't hear us properly.

Afterwards, participants swapped emails on what they thought was going on. Andrew explained that, while the furin cleavage site was arresting, his hunch was that the virus acquired it in an intermediate host species before jumping into humans.

The next day I gathered everyone's thoughts, including people like Michael Farzan, and emailed Tony and Francis:

On a spectrum if 0 is nature and 100 is release – I am honestly at 50! My guess is that this will remain grey, unless there is access to the Wuhan lab – and I suspect that is unlikely!

We agreed it had to be looked at quickly and forensically, ideally under a WHO umbrella, but that did not materialise (the agency was taken up with the emergency response). So, after those initial conversations, five scientists came together to take an investigation forward: Kristian; Eddie; Andrew; Bob; and W. Ian Lipkin, a Columbia University virologist who, in addition to being a well known virus hunter and SARS veteran, was scientific adviser to the film *Contagion*. They resolved to undertake a fingertip search of the literature, rake through accumulating research on the virus, study the epidemiological data and scrutinise samples of the virus, all to detect the trace of an unseen hand

Despite his experience with Ebola and Zika, Kristian had never fronted such a pressured and sensitive investigation: 'I was battling with the idea that, having raised the alarm, I might end up being the person who proved this new virus came from a lab,' he says. 'And I didn't necessarily want to be that person, well-known across the world ... And I was thinking, how do we even do this? Am I supposed to call the FBI? What burden of proof were we looking for?

'This couldn't just be me fiddling around with my analyses and then saying, "Yeah, it came from a lab" or "No, this virus is probably natural." When you make big claims like that, you had better be sure that you can conclude something based on evidence and not on speculation.' The matter was so sensitive that, apart from a handful of senior colleagues, his lab companions did not know what he was working on.

I included a reference to the conversations in a circular to select Wellcome colleagues afterwards:

You may have read in social media and others asking what the origins of this virus were. Very difficult to work out and exquisitely sensitive. We are engaged with China, with scientists in Australia, EU, UK, USA and with the WHO on this.

❋ ❋ ❋

It was indeed imperative to engage with China. In that first weekend of February, as it became clear from everyone that the origins of the virus deserved closer inspection, I got in touch, via an impeccably connected American friend, with an old contact in China. Chen Zhu was China's minister of health between 2007 and 2013. Originally trained as a 'barefoot doctor'* in rural China, he studied in Paris, learned to speak several languages and become a celebrated haematologist, specialising in leukaemia treatments. He is, without doubt, one of the most remarkable people I have ever met. Zhu is respected globally for his work in ensuring China is plugged in scientifically to the rest of the world, regardless of what is happening politically.

The phone call to Zhu took place on a secure line around midnight, which seemed appropriate for what I wanted to talk to him about. We discussed the outbreak and how it would cause disruption on a global scale. I mentioned the rumours that the novel coronavirus could be the result of a lab accident, though it was too early to say much more. I just wanted to let him know that, of course, people would be

---

* In the late 1960s, Chairman Mao promoted the idea of 'barefoot doctors', villagers who underwent a short period of training and returned to their rural communities as village doctors, promoting prevention and offering basic treatment based on a mix of western and traditional medicines.

asking questions. If a man-made virus became the narrative, I told him, we would be in for some turbulence and I wanted to make sure there were links into China whatever the outcome. I wanted him to know that scientists were working to establish the truth – but with a resolutely open mind. As ever, he took the news calmly.

My American friend Marty Murphy also joined the conversation but on an urgent practical matter: he had collected donations from US companies to send to Wuhan, then at the terrible peak of its epidemic. The Chinese city was running out of personal protective equipment and the local airports were shut. Marty managed to pull together a miracle of global generosity and solidarity: 154 pallets of PPE donated by US companies, including the pharmaceutical giant Amgen, sent on a UPS MD-11 cargo jet to Shanghai. From there, the PPE was loaded on to two Chinese domestic carriers and flown into Wuhan. That the UPS plane was allowed in Chinese airspace at all is down to Zhu.

Together, Marty and Zhu made impossible things happen.

❈ ❈ ❈

The following month, after the addition of important new information, endless analyses, intense discussions and many sleepless nights, Kristian Andersen, Andrew Rambaut, Ian Lipkin, Eddie Holmes and Bob Garry were ready to pronounce on the origins of the novel coronavirus. On 17 March 2020, in a clear, short paper entitled 'The Proximal Origin of SARS-CoV-2', the researchers stated: 'Our analyses clearly show that SARS-CoV-2 is not a laboratory construct or a purposefully manipulated virus.'

To begin with, the paper, published in the journal *Nature Medicine*, noted the two features of the coronavirus that had sparked concern. First, the virus glues itself with suspicious enthusiasm to human cells – or, in the language of the paper, 'appears to be optimised for binding to the human cell receptor ACE2'.* The receptor binding domain (RBD) of the virus fits the ACE2 receptor like a hand in a glove.

Second, the virus is then able to gain entry to cells almost as if it had a key. That is because the spike protein, the piece of the virus that enables infection, features a distinctive furin cleavage site. That was the specific bit of the genome that had caused so much consternation. It allows the spike protein to be cleaved, or split, to start the infection process – like removing a key from a bunch in order to unlock a door. Similar sites are seen in virulent pathogens like the viruses that cause bird flu and Ebola.

But many things, the authors explained, did not make sense if this was an engineered virus. The new coronavirus attached itself to cells quite differently from SARS-CoV-1 – and was also unlike any of the known viruses used in gain of function research in labs. That rendered deliberate manipulation an implausible scenario. Why? A malevolent scientist is still a scientist – and the most methodical way of conjuring up a nightmare virus would be to take a virus that is already a known quantity, such as SARS-CoV-1, and crank up its infectivity using known methods.

Or, as Kristian puts it, somewhat bluntly: 'Scientists are lazy. If we want to make viruses in the lab, we follow recipes we've used for decades because we know they work. This virus bore no lab signature whatsoever.' That spoke to Marion's early observation: why would a scheming scientist not use a known virus?

---

* ACE2 (Angiotensin-converting enzyme 2) is present in many organs, including the lungs, heart, blood vessels, kidneys and liver. Among other functions, it helps to regulate blood pressure and inflammation.

Rather, SARS-CoV-2 looked like a malign gift from nature. The paper offered two pieces of circumstantial evidence: first, that a bat coronavirus called RaTG13 was 96 per cent genetically similar to SARSCoV-2 but differed in the receptor binding domain; and second, that coronaviruses featuring identical receptor binding domains had just been found in Malayan pangolins, known to be imported illegally into parts of China. In short, the paper showed that the ingredients for SARS-CoV-2 were out in the wild. They did not need to have escaped, or been unleashed, from a containment lab.

That tallied with Andrew's idea that he circulated after the conference call with Tony Fauci and Francis Collins: that the receptor binding domain, a crucial portion of the virus, might have originated in an as-yet-unidentified intermediate species between bats and humans.

The paper then offered two scenarios. In the first, a bat coronavirus crossed into an intermediate species – perhaps a pangolin – and underwent further mutations. This new virus, having gained the genetic capability to survive in a broader range of hosts than just bats, then jumped into humans.

The second scenario is that a precursor to the new coronavirus crossed the species barrier undetected into humans many times, potentially over months or even years. Each transmission shuffled the genetic deck slightly, mostly resulting in viruses that didn't go anywhere. Eventually, a combination of random biological changes and natural selection hit a sweet spot, conjuring up a form of the virus able to clinch a foothold in a human host and, critically, acquire the capacity to pass from one person to another.

It is a respectable guess that SARS-CoV-2 could have appeared in this way, as HIV did in the 1930s from chimpanzees. With its newly minted ability to infect and transmit between people, SARS-CoV-2 took off sufficiently to cause an observable outbreak in December 2019 (strange though it sounds, it can be really hard to spot an outbreak: it means first looking for a signal among the noise, such as a slew of unexplained pneumonias, and recognising it as sufficiently anomalous to dig further).

Just because the natural world provides all the ingredients for SARS-CoV-2 does not prove the virus did not come from a lab; it is impossible to prove a negative without access to lab documents. But the simplest explanation remains the likeliest: nature plus bad luck. 'We know how powerful biology can be,' Marion says.

When the paper by Kristian and co was published, Bill Gallaher, a microbiologist at Louisiana State University, commented on virological.org that the lack of a matching RNA sequence in the literature rendered a lab origin highly unlikely:

No known viral RNA sequence is the daddy of SARS-CoV-2. No match. If it doesn't fit, you must acquit. It is all bat guano.

❋ ❋ ❋

The paper has been accessed online more than 5 million times and, Kristian accepts, might end up being the defining paper of his career: 'We never set out to write a historic paper that would be one of the best-read ever. We thought that when it was published it would be mostly ignored, because, well, there's a pandemic. We wrote it because scientists wanted to know whether this virus came from a lab. Today, researchers can cite our paper and say, "This lot looked at it and they're the kind of people who know what they're doing." I'm really happy that we managed to do that.'

Unlike Kristian, I expected the paper to whip up attention. As the virus spread, I could see the blame game was shaping up into an explosive political issue. Without a serious scientific investigation, published at speed, the rumours were going to fuel ongoing trouble.

Other theories still circulate. The Wuhan Institute of Virology housed a sample of the closest virus, RaTG13. Given that one of the institute's aims is to sample bat-borne viruses, the coincidence is not surprising. However, there has been intense focus on the work of Shi Zhengli, a Chinese virologist known as the 'Bat Woman' because of her work on bat viruses at the WIV. In 2012, she visited a copper mine in Yunnan where six miners were sickened by a mystery respiratory disease with similar symptoms to Covid-19. Three of the miners later died. She and her team collected a host of viruses, including RaTG13, from that mine and others afterwards, but her conclusion was that the miners' illness had been caused by a fungus. She had been studying coronaviruses at the lab and there had been security concerns raised about the WIV by US diplomats.

Is it possible that an infected bat researcher at the institute unwittingly spread the disease in Wuhan? Andrew believes that the probability of accidental escape from a lab, through someone becoming infected and then going on to infect others, is 'vanishingly small. It would mean someone going out into the wild, collecting the one-in-a-million virus capable of infecting humans, bringing it back to the lab and then making a whole series of mistakes.'

Andrew explains: 'That's just one very specific way of going from bat viruses in nature to a human epidemic, whereas there are tens of thousands or even millions of exposures to bat viruses in the wild potentially over long periods of time in large geographical areas. If a human-infectious virus was out there, it is infinitely more likely that one of these very large numbers of contacts could have acquired it.'

Could RaTG13, a sample of which is known to have been at WIV, have been worked up into something capable of infecting humans and then leaked or released? Any scientist wanting to turn RaTG13, or similar, into SARS-CoV-2 would have needed to conduct 'serial passage' of the starting virus, repeatedly growing the virus in different conditions to mimic the process of evolution. It is almost impossible, Kristian says, to put bat viruses through this process in the lab. He has tried to culture bat viruses many times and failed. Unsurprisingly, bat viruses prefer bats to Petri dishes.

The chain of infection into humans does not need to be directly bat-to-human; it could have happened via another species. Pangolins are not the only species in the frame. SARS-CoV-2 infects animals like ferrets and mink (known as mustelids) as efficiently as it infects humans, raising the possibility of a wild or farmed animal being the stepping stone between bats and people.

A joint WHO/China report published in March 2021 on the origins of SARS-CoV-2 concluded that a laboratory accident or deliberate release was very unlikely. It suggested the two most probable scenarios are: a jump from the host species, likely bats, to humans via an intermediate species; or direct infection from the host species.

Marion Koopmans was part of the WHO team that went into China, looked at the (possibly incomplete) evidence that the Chinese government made available and co-authored the March 2021 report. A virus journeying from bats into people via pangolins, Marion says, is a 'credible hypothesis, in terms of what we see in emerging diseases. [Pangolins] are endangered but also a delicacy for locals and tourists, so there is a big market. They are being collected from a wider and wider geographical area along smuggling routes. It's really a textbook way of getting problems with viruses.'

Another scenario favoured by authorities in China is that SARS-CoV-2 virus was imported into China via frozen food supply chains. A handful of outbreaks with apparent links to food markets led China to screen 1.4 million samples of frozen food; around 30 had traces of the virus (though Marion says this could be surface contamination). The WHO then commissioned its own studies to see whether the virus could withstand the subzero temperatures.

Marion explains: 'It's typical to get viruses in food but with freezing you would expect to lose a lot of infectivity. The WHO studies showed *Bingo!* If you put virus on a fish and freeze it for three weeks, you can just grow the virus back. It's stable. Based on all those kinds of findings, we said, "OK, we cannot rule it out."'

A smoking gun, like the unambiguous link that Marion helped to discover between camels and Middle East respiratory virus, would help to settle the matter. It would mean finding an extremely close match to SARS-CoV-2 in either nature or a lab. Andrew Rambaut speculates there may be a bat virus somewhere out there that is a closer match to SARS-CoV-2 than RaTG13. That might fill the gap in understanding the origins of this pandemic virus.

One reason why rumours persist is that the WHO delegation to China, which Marion joined, included Peter Daszak from the EcoHealth Alliance. The non-profit research organisation has funded research at the Wuhan Institute of Virology and Daszak had previously dismissed the idea of a lab origin for SARS-CoV-2. Even though he is an accomplished scientist, it would have been better for him to have recused himself and for the WHO to have appointed someone who would have been perceived as more impartial.

In May 2021, several scientists including Ralph Baric, one of the world's leading coronavirus researchers at the University of North Carolina, and Jesse Bloom, whose Seattle lab has been at the forefront of studying mutations, wrote a letter to the journal *Science* asking for a fresh investigation and demanding that labs, including the Wuhan Institute of Virology, open their books and documentation to outsiders. Soon after, President Biden also requested a fresh look at the evidence.

We need to know where this virus came from, especially if we want to prevent something similar happening in the future. So we should continue looking for answers – and hope that new evidence comes to light. There is, though, no guarantee that we will find the evidence we seek, nor any certainty that we will understand how the outbreak started. As things currently stand, the evidence strongly suggests that Covid-19 arose after a natural spillover event, but nobody is yet in a position to rule out an alternative. In the meantime, we should be reducing the chances of future spillovers and making sure labs are safe and transparent in their work.

❋ ❋ ❋

The intense drama around the origins question made me stop and think about the biases we all bring to the table, the kind of biases that feed conspiracy theories. Mine was seeing a peculiar feature in the virus and wondering why it had started in Wuhan, a city known for its lab. I had put two and two together and made five.

Kristian admits to having his own biases too, which took a proper scientific analysis to overturn: 'I look back now and think, man, there was a lot of stuff we didn't know. Like just how prevalent the features that worried us were; how they come and go all the time in coronaviruses and there's nothing mysterious about them. One huge bias was only comparing the new virus to SARS-CoV-1. Because SARS-CoV-1 didn't share these odd features, we assumed something mysterious was going on. That's not how evolution works.'

The tragedy is that this entire controversy over the origins of the pandemic coronavirus turned out to be a distraction. The Trump administration, which demanded that the US National Academy of Medicine investigate, threw so much energy and effort into finger-pointing that it failed to adequately prepare for the pandemic. The conspiracist blame game was a fig leaf to disguise the failure of American governance.

By early February, the new virus was causing havoc and geopolitical tensions everywhere, including in international waters. On 5 February 2020, the *Diamond Princess*, a luxury cruise ship built for more than two thousand passengers and a crew of a thousand-plus, was quarantined in the Japanese port of Yokohama. The Japanese government instigated the drastic measure because an 80-year-old passenger from Hong Kong had disembarked on 25 January and subsequently tested positive. By 21 February, 634 people on board had tested positive.

The docked vessel became a hotbed of transmission and a staple of international news bulletins. It focused minds on the still-complex issue of how to balance public health with global justice. Passengers, running short of medicines and patience, were pleading to be allowed to leave. Countries sent charter planes to rescue nationals from the plague ship and protested at their incarceration. There was confusion over who was supposed to manage the crisis: Japanese officials, the ship's captain or the company that owned the ship.

It was a tragic situation not just for passengers but for the crew: four to a bathroom, lacking the facilities to isolate if they fell ill, and working across the whole vessel to keep it functioning. At the lowest point of the crisis, the *Diamond Princess* accounted for the largest cluster of cases outside mainland China.

The ship was also a contained environment that allowed some of the disease's characteristics to be teased out. One of its key contributions was to confirm the role of asymptomatic people in spreading the virus: at first, people without symptoms were not tested. When the policy was changed to universal testing, it revealed that, by 20 February according to the medical journal *Eurosurveillance*, around 18 per cent of those infected showed no symptoms. Cruises attract an older clientele; it was reasonable to assume an even higher proportion of people showing no symptoms in the general population.

In mid-February, a contact in the US sent me a back-of-the-envelope calculation of how the epidemic might play out in the US, based in part on the epidemiological information emerging from the *Diamond Princess*. Assuming a population of 325 million and an attack rate of 30 per cent, the guess-timates were horrifying: 98 million people falling sick, 12 million hospitalised, two million in intensive care and between 300,000 and 1,000,000 deaths over the course of a year.

These figures, sadly, were closer to the ballpark than President Trump's analysis in March 2020 that the virus 'will disappear'. By 22 February 2021, a year after the *Diamond Princess* episode, there had been 28 million confirmed cases in the US and more than 500,000 deaths.

※ ※ ※

In 2016, following the record Ebola epidemic in West Africa, the World Health Organization decided it needed a strategy and preparedness plan, to guide research activities in the event of future shocks. Four of us – WHO assistant director general Marie-Paule Kieny; Ana-Maria Henao-Restrepo, a WHO specialist in vaccines; Mike Ryan, director of the WHO's Health Emergencies Programme; and me – set up something called the WHO R&D Blueprint, that would bring together scientists, public health specialists and regulators in an emergency to fast-track research into diagnostics, treatments and vaccines. Its first achievement was the Merck vaccine against Ebola, which came out of trials in Guinea during the epidemic. It was an incredible validation of what a mix of strategy and speed could pull off: a first-ever vaccine for a disease delivered in the middle of a catastrophic epidemic.

In the perpetual tussle between people and pathogens, the Blueprint would become part of the battle plan. Other critical legacies from the previous outbreak, and now part of that battle plan, include CEPI (Coalition for Epidemic Preparedness Innovations), set up to finance and coordinate vaccine efforts; and ISARIC (International Severe Acute Respiratory and emerging Infection Consortium), which allows standardised clinical data to be collected and shared in public health emergencies. Both have revolutionised the speed at which things can happen. By the third week of January 2020, when scientists were still discussing whether this new virus could pass between people, CEPI was signing agreements with vaccine companies like Moderna; and ISARIC had swung into action in Wuhan. These three additions to the global health armamentarium – the WHO R&D Blueprint, CEPI and ISARIC – are particular achievements that I am proud to be associated with.

On 11 and 12 February 2020, the WHO held its first R&D Blueprint meeting on the novel coronavirus, bringing together at least 500 people in Geneva, in person and remotely, to set the scientific agenda for what would need to be done, both for understanding the disease itself and developing countermeasures, such as diagnostic tests, drugs and vaccines.

I ended up arriving late. I had committed, for environmental reasons, not to fly if travelling in Europe and, after leaving Lyon, my train got stuck just outside Geneva. It was a little embarrassing: I was co-chairing the meeting with Marie-Paule and joined after a coffee break.

It seems remarkable now, but it seemed as if the world was there in the grand main hall at the WHO HQ. Tedros was there. George Gao, head of China CDC, joined by video. Doctors from Wuhan and elsewhere in China turned up in person or remotely. People from all over the world, and in social sciences, ethics, virology and immunology, were represented. Countries sent diplomats from their missions in Geneva. There was a poignant absence: Peter Salama, until 2019 a key figure in the WHO's Health Emergencies Programme. Peter, who I spent a lot of time with during the Ebola crisis, died suddenly in late January, aged just 51.

By the time of that first Blueprint meeting, approaching mid-February, people were just starting to grasp the scale of the epidemic in China and surrounding countries. I had compiled a bullet-point list on this unknown disease and circulated it to a few Wellcome colleagues before leaving for Geneva:

Estimates on

Incubation period (time from being infected to symptoms) – 3–10 days

Infectious period (time you can pass it on to someone else) – 1–10 days

Infectious with very mild symptoms – sore throat, mild cough, headache (possibly asymptomatic) through to very severe.

R0 estimates – 2.5–3.0

These are extraordinary characteristics for a novel pathogen for which we have no immunity

In China, Case Fatality Rate (CFR) is likely >10% ...

Estimate now that there are perhaps 200,000–300,000 people who have been or are infected in Hubei Province ...

To give you an idea of the pressure hospitals in Wuhan are under – the number of patients with severe disease is increasing by an order of magnitude every 7 days.

A 1000 bed hospital has been built in a week and gymnasiums have been turned into additional hospitals…

Few reports yet in children not clear why ...

Increasing number of healthcare workers becoming ill.

These estimates obviously have serious consequences – they are closer to UK reasonable worst case scenario for planning of a pandemic.

The case fatality rate (CFR) is the proportion of confirmed cases that end in death within a certain time period. R0 (or R-nought), refers to the basic reproduction number, which represents how quickly a disease spreads without any interventions (such as social distancing or masks). An R0 of 3 meant each infected person was passing it to three others on average. In turn, those three would spread it to another nine in total; those nine to another 27. That is the nature of exponential spread.

That WHO R&D Blueprint Meeting put the agency at the centre of the global response and served as the catalyst that got the world moving: the sharing of samples; more companies starting vaccine work; the kick-starting of networked clinical trials across the world that would allow us to pool findings on potential treatments. That meeting, plus the sense of urgency that many of us had radiated at Davos, was why we got Covid-19 diagnostics, treatments, vaccines in less than a year.

❋ ❋ ❋

'Are you a spy?' asked the taxi driver, as I jumped into his cab at Munich airport on Friday 14 February 2020. I was on my way to the Munich Security Conference, which takes place in one of the city's hotels every year and, with its focus on global security, seems to draw an even more exclusive crowd than Davos. Panellists that year included Nancy Pelosi, Justin Trudeau, Emmanuel Macron and Jens Stoltenberg, NATO's secretary general. For the past five years, I have attended it every February, and my first-hand experience of the controversy over the origins of the new coronavirus made my 2020 trip to Munich feel especially relevant.

Outside the hotel, there are always a lot of big men walking round in uniform wearing earpieces, and black cars lining up to deliver important-looking people. Inside, it is how I imagine the Silk Road to have been, a melting pot with people of all nationalities rubbing shoulders. I just wander around amused by the fact that the Iranian spies and the American spies are meeting for coffee (at least, I assume they are spies). It's almost exclusively male.

It is not the sort of conference to which you can blag an invitation. Mine came through Sam Nunn, the Democratic senator who set up the Nuclear Threat Initiative, which has since broadened its remit to look at other security threats, including biosecurity. I got in touch with Sam a few years ago because I felt that the world was highly vulnerable to emerging risks and threats from nature, and that we scientists could learn something from the spies. In 2014, for example, we jointly ran a tabletop exercise at Munich simulating the deliberate release of a pathogen. Wellcome has teamed up on projects with organisations like the NTI ever since.

A nuclear or terrorist threat is very much like the challenge we face in public health and epidemiology: seeing the signal for the noise. How do we sift through millions of events to identify the ones that matter? How do we respond immediately to a biological threat to potentially prevent a pandemic? It is not that easy, in practice, to spot early outbreaks of a new disease.

That difficulty is compounded by the inability to go into countries and look for biological threats in the way that agencies can demand access to countries to search for chemical or nuclear weapons. I am not sure any country would allow such an investigation. Another parallel between terrorism and biosecurity is the variety of actors who can stir up trouble: technological advances mean that big states and rich institutions no longer have a monopoly on building either bombs or bioweapons. The counterpart of the lone gunman could be a hobbyist genetically modifying viruses in her garage.

Maintaining a scientific presence in the security world also achieves another end: making sure that decisions on dual-use technology, such as the gain of function research that scientists like Ron Fouchier practise, are not monopolised or controlled by the security community. Dual-use technology, like the techniques to make viruses more contagious or deadly, can seem very scary. But shutting them down would mean critical science, needed for threat surveillance and safety, not being done or being carried out under the radar. We need to be more nuanced and pragmatic about it.

At Munich, I met with Sam, as well as Ernest Moniz, who served as Obama's Energy Secretary. We talked a lot about the new coronavirus. I was rattling on at length about how worrying it was and laying out where I thought the epidemic was heading. The virus itself was not news to them but the depth of concern in the global health community was.

By then, in mid-February, very few people in the US had grasped how fast things were moving. Even at Munich, among the very community tasked with spotting black swans, the crises that spring from nowhere, the coronavirus outbreak was gliding towards them relatively unchecked. Certainly, the White House was nowhere near assigning it the seriousness it merited. It is fair to say it was in denial.

※ ※ ※

Straight after the conference, I caught the train from Munich to Salzburg. This is part of the Farrar family's annual routine: I travel from Munich, which is usually just before the February half-term, to meet Christiane and the children, who fly in from the UK. We then head to a little village called Hinterstoder in the mountains.

We have been going there to ski for about 20 years, and started taking the kids as toddlers. This time it was four of us rather than five, as our eldest son, Sam, was at college. We always head to the same farm: on top of a mountain with just ten simple rooms and no through road. It is unbelievably beautiful. The owners have become family friends, a link that deepened after a skiing accident there in 2015 put me in hospital for two nights.

It was supposed to be a week off, but of course that was never going to happen. This was a very intense time. There were so many phone calls: with Eddie and Kristian about the origins paper (then yet to be published), conversations with Peter Horby and Bin Cao, a doctor in China, on the clinical studies they had set up in Wuhan, an important piece of the WHO Blueprint plan. It wasn't much of a holiday and I barely hit the slopes.

By this time, the new virus was spreading quietly across Europe. Researchers would later count more than 1,300 separate occasions when the virus was seeded into the UK, mostly in February and March. The kindling for the UK's epidemic was not flying in from China but from elsewhere in Europe. It was being innocently imported by families like ours, fresh from half-term skiing trips in snowy northern Italy; others brought it back weeks later from sunshine breaks in Spain and France.

Spring was in the air and thousands of chains of transmission were being sparked across Europe.

4

Worrying about a ripple ... [*]

25 FEBRUARY 2020

Known cases: 80,239
China: 77,780 cases, 2,666 deaths
2,459 cases in 33 other countries, 34 deaths
UK cases: 13

WHEN I GOT BACK FROM AUSTRIA, it was time
to catch up with what was happening in the UK. On 25
February 2020, I attended my first SAGE meeting in person.
The Scientific Advisory Group for Emergencies (SAGE) is an
ad-hoc group of scientists and experts across universities and
industry invited to offer scientific advice on specific crises
either taking place in the UK or forecast to have a significant
impact on the country.

Up until then, with the epidemic centred on China and its
neighbours, and the international plan for emergency research
taking priority, I had joined intermittently by phone. I also
had my own backchannel with two other SAGE advisers, both
of them infectious disease epidemiologists whom I respect

---

[*]   'It's like worrying about a ripple when there's a fucking tsunami heading straight
for you.' John Edmunds, London School of Hygiene and Tropical Medicine

hugely as colleagues: John Edmunds from the London School of Hygiene and Tropical Medicine and Neil Ferguson, from London's Imperial College. I met John many years ago at a typhoid conference in Fiji, and I first met Neil when I was dealing with H5N1 bird flu in Vietnam. Both are outstanding scientists who had helped to model pandemic flu preparedness plans more than a decade earlier.

Technically, SAGE is a subcommittee of COBR (Civil Contingencies Committee), sometimes called COBRA*. This committee is brought together by the government to handle large-scale emergencies, such as natural disasters, disease outbreaks and industrial accidents. It does not publish minutes and neither did SAGE early in the coronavirus outbreak.

SAGE has convened eight times since 2009 and I had sat on it before in 2014, during the Ebola epidemic in West Africa. The group is usually chaired by whoever is the UK government's chief scientific adviser at the time. Patrick Vallance took on the role in 2018 and could never have dreamed he was signing up for the worst health crisis in living memory. He trained as a doctor and taught at University College London before heading research and development at GlaxoSmith-Kline. We have known each other for about eight years, as long as I have been director of the Wellcome Trust.

I had already texted both Patrick and Chris Whitty (the UK government's chief medical adviser) back in January to share my concerns: that this was a coronavirus related to SARS; that human-to-human transmission was possible, as well as asymptomatic transmission; and that there had already been geographical spread.

Patrick had arranged the very first 'precautionary' meeting of SAGE on 22 January 2020, to which I had dialled in. Neil,

---

* COBR stands for Cabinet Office Briefing Room, where the committee convenes.

who had also been involved in the early WHO response, had been quick off the mark in calculating the true size of the outbreak: by 16 January he had deduced, based on exported cases, that Wuhan was harbouring 1,000-plus cases by 6 January, more than ten times the official figure. A group of Mandarin-speaking PhD students at Imperial was scraping information from national and provincial government websites in China, and from preprint papers.

On Friday 24 January, Neil, who guessed that some infected travellers were slipping through the net, emailed me, Patrick and Chris to say that 'NHS preparedness should be kicked up a gear.' We had also had that very important conference call on 27 January, launching UK research into vaccines and therapies into the so-called Wuhan coronavirus.

Patrick took our worries seriously because he knows my background in emerging infections. He knew I would not overplay something that was not worth worrying about. There was no human immunity to this new pathogen; this was a respiratory disease spreading, in some cases asymptomatically, in a big urban centre in winter; Chinese New Year was fast approaching and there were no diagnostic tests, treatments or vaccines. There were no vaccines for any member of the coronavirus family of viruses.

I've known Chris for years too: he also trained in infectious diseases and did a period of study in Vietnam. The global health and infectious disease community can sometimes adopt a slightly weary attitude of 'We've seen it all before and these things are never as bad as you think.' And that was Chris, initially: he wanted to be much more cautious, to wait and weigh everything before taking action. The lesson from every epidemic is that if you wait until you know everything, then you are too late. If you fall behind an epidemic curve, it is extraordinarily hard to get back in front of it.

The UK, meanwhile, was clocking up its first known cases in January 2020: a woman who returned from Hubei province on 23 January subsequently developed fever, sore throat and dry cough. A household contact later developed symptoms, suggesting person-to-person transmission. Both were hospitalised in Newcastle, in north-east England, on 31 January as a precaution and discharged after a mild illness.

That friction, between waiting and wading in, led to a palpable tension between Patrick and Chris in the early weeks of 2020, particularly given the apparent absence of political leadership in that period. Boris Johnson, the prime minister, did not attend the first five COBR meetings on coronavirus in January and February 2020.

Chris, though, had more experience than Patrick of operating in political circles: he was in government in 2009, during the H1N1 swine flu pandemic. It was projected to lead to 65,000 deaths; in the event, there were fewer than 300. Dame Sally Davies, then England's chief medical officer, was unfairly criticised for overreacting. The UK stockpiled oseltamivir (sold as Tamiflu) and other measures at great expense.

That backlash possibly made Chris wary of the same happening this time round. He talked about the outbreak as a marathon not a sprint. In a sense, outbreaks *are* marathons, but there are times in every long-distance race when you need to go fast. That go-slow outlook pervaded much of the thinking in January and February 2020 in the UK, even though all the information that had accumulated by the end of January should have set off the loudest of sirens.

✻ ✻ ✻

SAGE collects and analyses scientific evidence to inform, not set, government policy. The group draws, in turn, from the wisdom of multiple subgroups that feed existing and specially commissioned research into its deliberations. By 25 February 2020, when I started attending the Westminster meetings in person, those subgroups were already hard at work. Among them were the Scientific Pandemic Influenza Group on Modelling (SPI-M), on which both John and Neil sit; the Scientific Pandemic Insights Group on Behaviours (SPI-B); and the New and Emerging Respiratory Virus Threats Advisory Group (NERVTAG), which John and Neil also attend. NERVTAG is chaired by Peter Horby, with whom I worked in Vietnam on H5N1 and who, together with Martin Landray, has pioneered lifesaving studies into potential treatments for Covid-19 in the RECOVERY trial.

There were also subgroups covering genomics, crucial for monitoring new variants, and health data, as well as ethics. There were observers from the Prime Minister's office, usually Ben Warner or occasionally Dominic Cummings. Public Health England and the NHS were always represented.

Adding in the chief scientists and other emissaries for various government departments, plus the devolved nations, I would guess that SAGE has between 200 and 300 people to call on in total, although there were rarely more than 20 to 30 in attendance (plus others dialling in on often ropey lines). I do not recall Treasury officials at the meetings I attended. Outsiders were occasionally invited in; at one meeting I sat next to Demis Hassabis, a researcher who cofounded artificial intelligence start-up DeepMind.

The SAGE meetings mostly took place in a basement at 10 Victoria Street in Westminster, which also houses the Government Office for Science. We would go through security and head downstairs through corridors with peeling paint. Then we would swipe our security passes to access a waiting area, strewn with unwashed cups that looked like they had been there for weeks. Finally, we would stream into the cavernous meeting room with the huge table in the middle, around which we all took a seat according to where our name badges were placed. We were so focused on the matter in hand that I cannot even remember whether the room had windows.

* * *

Looking back, the minutes of SAGE meetings[*] up until 25 February 2020 paint a portrait of the UK shuffling towards a precipice. On 28 January, they record that the epidemic in Wuhan was doubling every three to four days, and that asymptomatic transmission was a possibility. On 3 February, masks came under scrutiny: there was no evidence that they prevented wearers from infection but early hints that masks worn by infected people could help to cut spread. Any small benefit, though, might be outweighed by the risk of a resulting mask shortage for health workers.

By 15 February, the outbreak in China was seen as uncontainable, according to the minutes. On 18 February, it was minuted that Public Health England could perhaps cope with five coronavirus cases a week, generating 800 contacts that would need tracing. That could be scaled up to 50 cases a week and 8,000 contacts – but, if sustained transmission took off, contact tracing would become unviable. Today, it seems unbelievable that, thanks to a decade of austerity, the world's fifth richest economy would be so woefully poised to respond and scale up fast to a public health emergency. The

---

[*]   SAGE minutes were initially kept secret but, following pressure from Patrick
       Vallance, Chris Whitty, SAGE advisers and some MPs, the government changed
       policy on 29 May 2020. On that day, it also released minutes of the 34 SAGE
       meetings that had already happened.

running down of public health in the decade before 2020 helped to turn what would have been a serious challenge into an ongoing tragedy.

On 20 February, SAGE sought clarity on what the government was trying to achieve by managing the outbreak: flattening the peak, spreading the duration of any epidemic or avoiding a winter epidemic? SAGE was explicitly seeking strategic direction from Number 10, so it could advise on what actions were needed to achieve them.

The malaise was disquieting, given that both Neil and John feared that chains of transmission might already be underway. It felt as if there might only be a small window to act, but nobody had bothered to open it. John was asking me and Neil whether it would be feasible for the army to open field hospitals and bring nurses out of retirement. Those were not the kind of questions that SAGE advisers were supposed to tackle – and we soon we began to worry that nobody else was tackling them either.

At the 25 February SAGE meeting, we discussed a paper that looked at whether four measures could put the brakes on an epidemic: closing universities and schools; getting people to isolate at home if they suspected they were infected (home isolation); quarantining entire households if one person became infected (household quarantine); and social distancing.

These are called non-pharmaceutical interventions (NPIs) and, later on, behavioural and social interventions (BSIs). They are the first steps towards what we now know as lockdown, although we never used that word at the time.

The modelling showed that combining multiple measures could realistically slow the spread, simply because they cut social contact. Our advice was that any such steps, if taken, should be combined, and mandatory not optional. You cannot tell people to stay home only if they feel like it.

That paper, signed off by the SPI-M modelling group, also contained a reference to the established concept of herd immunity, sometimes called population immunity (I prefer the latter). Herd immunity has come to mean different things to different people, especially since early January 2020, but it has a specific meaning in epidemiology: it brings an epidemic to an end. If enough people in the population become immune to a contagious disease, they become dead ends for the disease. Transmission should fall or stop. As John explains: 'There is only one way an epidemic like this ends, and that's with herd immunity, achieved either with or without vaccines. That's it. If you don't have long-lasting immunity [from natural infection], the epidemic doesn't come to an end.'

The more transmissible a disease, the greater the proportion of the population that must be immune to stop it spreading. This percentage is called the herd immunity threshold; in March 2020, it was estimated at about 60 per cent for SARS-CoV-2 (it is closer to 95 per cent for measles, which is why childhood vaccination rates are watched so closely). Herd immunity has always, to my knowledge, been achieved through vaccination but, in theory at least, could also be reached through natural infection – providing that natural infection leads to long-lasting immunity. There is, however, no precedent in the modern era for populations achieving herd immunity to a novel disease through natural infection.

The modelling paper posited that 'aggressive NPIs' had the potential to slow the epidemic but there could be a rebound in infections once measures were lifted. The rebound meant the epidemic would ultimately claim the same number of casualties 'though if measures are fine-tuned to allow sufficient transmission to allow population immunity (acquired through infection) to reach the herd immunity threshold, significant reductions in overall attack are also possible'.

That phrase had the potential to be read as a point in favour of herd immunity by natural infection, even though the policy was never advocated by SAGE (for starters, it could not be assumed that people would acquire immunity if infected). Herd immunity would become a highly contested issue in the weeks to come.

Over the next three meetings, which I could not attend, those NPIs came in for further scrutiny. The lockdowns in China, Hong Kong and Singapore seemed to be having an effect: their epidemics were slowing, with China already seemingly past its peak. In Hong Kong and Vietnam, remarkably, no healthcare workers had become infected.

The minutes, though, revealed that SAGE was wary of giving lockdown the credit. Did we know that China was sharing all its data and that its numbers really were dropping? If so, was it thanks to these extreme measures, the Wuhan lockdown, rather than to some unknown feature of the new virus? Could the epidemic be waning because the virus had swept through the population and was now hitting a wall of immunity?

Even if a lockdown worked in a country like China, could you pull it off in the UK? Could any government in Western Europe really tell people, 'You can't leave your house'? At the end of February 2020, there was almost a disbelief, including from me, that it was possible. We know differently now. Even though I had lived in Vietnam for nearly two decades, I wish SAGE had drawn on a wider group of experts with first-hand insights from China and the surrounding region.

There were other potential drawbacks of enacting some NPIs: measures would hit hardest those in precarious work or on low incomes, and the vulnerable – and, back in March 2020, nobody knew when, or even if, a vaccine would arrive. On top of that, shutting down society might be the equivalent of coiling a spring, leading to an enormous wave of infection when released. This might push a spring-to-summer wave of illness into autumn and winter, when the National Health Service would be at its most fragile because of winter pressures from flu and other seasonal illnesses.

I did not agree with postponing actions or interventions on the basis of a possible rebound: it amounted to accepting a huge number of deaths now in the uncertain hope of avoiding an unknown number of deaths later, an unethically unjustifiable trade-off. Postponing infections might actually save lives, because the delay reduces transmission and buys time to put other measures in place. Even if telling people to stay home in March risked causing a winter wave, it would have afforded a breathing space for the government to: organise more hospital beds and ventilators; increase testing and contact tracing; order protective equipment; marshal research into the virus; enable clinicians to develop plans for treatment; and bring effective drugs and vaccines closer to fruition.

John agrees that fretting about winter pressures felt like the wrong priority: 'It seemed so ridiculous. It's like worrying about a ripple on the surface of the sea when there's a fucking tsunami out in the bay heading straight for you.'

❁ ❁ ❁

On 3 March, the government sprang a surprise: the Coronavirus Action Plan. The plan had four phases: contain, delay, research and mitigate. The aim was to first contain the cases that cropped up by finding infected people (through testing), isolating them and tracing their contacts; if that failed to stop spread, there would be an attempt to delay any epidemic into the summer, using measures that people could take themselves, such as hand-washing and a 'catch it, bin it, kill it' approach to coughs and sneezes, as well as as-yet-unspecified measures still being discussed by advisers (in reality, the NPIs like home quarantine and household isolation). The social impacts of such measures, the plan stated, would be balanced against their possible benefits.

Research had started into tests and vaccines (the UK gave an initial £20m to CEPI, the Coalition for Epidemic Preparedness Innovations, for vaccines). Should the outbreak worsen, the focus would move to mitigation, providing hospital care for the sickest and community support for those ill at home. The great majority of people, the plan noted, would have 'a mild-to-moderate, but self-limiting illness – similar to seasonal flu'.

Neil explains that, in the models of how the disease would spread, mitigation was synonymous with the acquisition of herd immunity: 'It meant we weren't trying to stop something. Mitigation means slowing the spread a bit, so you try to reduce mortality, but the aim is not to stop the epidemic in its tracks. You do reduce the number of people infected, but the aim is to get the epidemic over with.' It is distinct from suppression, which means trying to stop spread in the first place. Mitigation and suppression are captured distinctly in epidemiological modelling: suppression indicates a strategy to keep R below 1, to shrink the epidemic; in mitigation, R can rise above 1, representing a spreading epidemic.

Boris Johnson certainly did not sound as if he wanted to stop the epidemic in its tracks. He was clear to the nation, as he presented the Coronavirus Action Plan, that 'for the vast majority of the people of this country, we should be going about our business as usual'.

John was surprised at the announcement: 'I went back to the minutes to see if we had ever properly discussed that four-phase strategy. The answer was no. The politicians came up with that strategy and our job was to make it work.' Neil, too, felt the plan simply codified a strategy that was already in train.

Likening Covid-19 to seasonal flu seemed an oddly hands-off approach to a virus that so many other countries were taking extremely seriously. By looking at data from multiple sources, such as from the *Diamond Princess* cruise ship, Neil and John had arrived at their own estimates of the reproduction number and case fatality rate (CFR – the ratio of confirmed deaths to confirmed diagnoses over a particular period). R was between 2 and 3; the CFR was maybe 2–3 per cent. A virus of that pathogenicity, or clinical severity, would claim colossal casualties if left to circulate. Even with a CFR of 1 per cent, it would mean 1 in 100 of identified cases would die. That made it around ten times deadlier than seasonal flu.

Says John: 'All our initial suspicions and fears about the coronavirus, which we had used to model reasonable worst-case scenarios, were being confirmed week by week, day by day. To all intents and purposes, this coronavirus looked very much like the pandemic flu* that everyone had been war-gaming with for years. Frankly, it looked pretty bad. It stacked up to half a million deaths.'

The trouble was, the virus was already circulating. On 5 March came news of 115 known cases in the UK, and the country's first coronavirus death, of a woman in her 70s who had recently tested positive for the virus. She had not been abroad.†

---

*   A new flu virus to which there is no human immunity.

†   It has since been reported that an 84-year-old man died in hospital in southern England on 30 January 2020, and it was only months later that coronavirus was detected in tissue samples. That would suggest the disease had been circulating for longer than initially assumed, and presumably spread further.

Those cases, we all knew, were the visible tip of an enormous iceberg, with at least hundreds and more likely thousands beneath an outwardly calm surface. Containment, the first stage of the government plan, was evidently off the table.

It was time to move to 'delay'.

※ ※ ※

The next day, Friday 6 March 2020, I received a tearful phone call from a contact in the charity Médecins sans Frontières (Doctors Without Borders). She was calling not from a conflict zone, or from a devastating natural disaster in a remote part of the Global South. She was dialling from northern Italy – watching the healthcare system of a G7 country fall apart. SARS-CoV-2 had arrived in Italy with a vengeance. There were more patients needing ventilation, she sobbed, than machines available. What had happened to China was now materialising in Europe.

That weekend, I included the bare bones of her dispatch in my confidential update to Wellcome colleagues:

I spoke with MSF-Italy on Friday night and they fear that the health system in Italy is close to collapse. Two weeks ago, Italy had 76 cases, it now has >7500 confirmed cases and with a rise from 233 deaths on Saturday to 366 on Sunday. As you will have seen on the news, Italy has now quarantined over a quarter of the population in the north of the country. The health, social, economic and political consequences of this are totally unknown.

Italy, which cordoned off northern regions from late February, put a national lockdown in place on 9 March. I had already called Tim Cook in Bath, so he could get the word out to intensive care networks across the country.

The dire situation in northern Italy focused minds in the next SAGE meeting on Tuesday 10 March. I relayed chilling status reports from my contacts there. It was battlefield medicine, deciding who to save and who to leave to die. Doctors were traumatised at having to choose who to put on the last ventilator. This wasn't China, or Korea, or any other country five thousand miles away. This was a sophisticated, rich country on our doorstep, and the health service was collapsing.

The UK was heading down the same terrible path: the country was already more stricken than anyone had realised and about to be hit with, literally, a wave of devastation. My attitude was changing too: if Italy had no option but to copy China, the UK would have to follow suit. I would have to question my own prejudices about what was possible or acceptable. I believe that what happened in Italy, and its decision to copy China in locking down, altered the course of the pandemic in Western Europe and radically changed attitudes in this country.

Epidemics tend to follow a curve that is shaped by how transmissible the disease is. Plotted against time, the line starts rising almost imperceptibly, as one case becomes two or three, and two become four or six. For a highly transmissible disease, it does not take long for the gradient to tick upwards sharply, as numbers rise exponentially* to a peak

---

* A quantity rises 'exponentially' when its rate of change is dependent on the quantity itself. Think of it like a person spreading a disease: if Patient Zero infects three people, and those three go on to infect another nine, and then those nine infect another 27, each generation of infection encompasses significantly more people. That is why graphs of Covid-19 infections plotted over time start slowly but climb rapidly. This is the reason that experts advocate early intervention to stop spread.

before falling again and tailing off because people change their behaviour or the population acquires herd immunity, limiting further spread.

Judging by what was happening elsewhere, Wuhan had passed the peak, Italy was rising to a crescendo and, chillingly, the UK was only about four to five weeks behind Italy. We knew this thanks to another shocking fact disclosed at that 10 March SAGE meeting: surveillance had belatedly revealed between 5,000 and 10,000 cases across the UK.

As sure as night followed day, it would only be a matter of days or weeks before infections turned into illness, hospitalisations and deaths. The peak, the modellers warned, could come the following month, if no action was taken. In the coming weeks it would be Britons, not Italians, gasping for high-flow oxygen. Those 5,000 to 10,000 newly infected individuals were still out in their communities, touching off further chains of transmission.

In terms of the Coronavirus Action Plan, we were well beyond 'delay' but the 'mitigation' plans looked dangerously inadequate. Operationally, the UK was desperately behind the curve. Public Health England was looking at being able to ramp up to a few hundred tests a day, even though the epidemic would be growing by thousands every few days. There was barely any discussion about NHS capacity. Bed occupancy was already tight, but there were no forward projections of what might be needed in terms of beds and ventilators.

As March wore on, I was surprised that Simon Stevens, the chief executive of the NHS who has since announced his retirement, did not attend SAGE, though Stephen Powis, its clinical director, did join. A gap was opening up between the advice coming from SAGE and the healthcare provision needed. That gap was worsened by the time lags built into a creaking system with many moving parts: it takes time to turn advice into action, and longer still for action to have an impact. Those lags are disastrous when an epidemic is doubling every few days.

It was not within SAGE's remit to advise on operational matters like bed capacity or the supply of personal protective equipment to healthcare workers, and we all understood that; it wasn't our area of expertise. John, however, who can be quite intense, took it upon himself to constantly push against that constraint. He devised his own deliberate behavioural strategy in SAGE meetings, which was to look political advisers directly in the eye while repeating the phrase, 'We are talking about hundreds of thousands of deaths.' He just wanted a reaction, an acknowledgement, that those in power understood what was coming.

Neil felt similarly: he had spent the first two weeks of March 2020 modelling, at the request of the Cabinet Office and Number 10, multiple scenarios that invariably ended up with deaths running into six figures: 'I never felt it was my view to say what policy government should adopt but I was slightly incredulous. There seemed to be a disconnect between all the effort being put into analysing these policy options and any understanding of what it would actually look like if that sort of thing happened.'

One widespread frustration was that only some modelling scenarios were getting through to decision-makers. Perfectly sensible central estimates were being touted as reasonable worst-case scenarios, as happened after a meeting between modellers and NHS analysts at Imperial College on 1 March 2020, held to project future healthcare demand. Neil says: 'It was a frustration to me that [our numbers] were presented as the reasonable worst case, because the very use of those words means it's viewed somehow as being unlikely. There was an intrinsic conservatism and a disbelief that this could ever happen.'

Something must have percolated through, however. Number 10 advisers Ben Warner and Dominic Cummings showed signs of increasing unease at the SAGE meetings they attended. Patrick Vallance was becoming anxious, too.

And then herd immunity stampeded on to the scene. It caused a public outcry.

❋ ❋ ❋

David Halpern, the head of the Behavioural Insights team at Number 10 (often called the 'nudge unit'), was at the 10 March SAGE meeting. On the same day, he told BBC News: 'There's going to be a point, assuming the epidemic flows and grows, as we think it probably will do, where you'll want to cocoon, you'll want to protect those at-risk groups so they basically don't catch the disease, and by the time they come out of their cocooning herd immunity's been achieved in the rest of the population.' This was never the view of SAGE.

The day after, Boris Johnson told breakfast television that one possible strategy was 'perhaps to take [the virus] on the chin, take it all in one go and allow the disease … to move through the population, without taking as many draconian measures'.

Patrick gave an interview in which he said: 'Our aim is to try to reduce the peak, broaden the peak, not suppress it completely; also, because the vast majority of people get a mild illness, to build up some kind of herd immunity so more people are immune to this disease and we reduce the transmission, at the same time we protect those who are most vulnerable to it.'

It surprised me when I later heard of these comments mentioned in media interviews and press conferences. Herd immunity via natural infection was not something that I recall being explicitly recommended by SAGE or even discussed at SAGE meetings as a strategy. Other advisers share this recollection.

Herd immunity by natural infection is a possible consequence, a potential outcome, of a disease spreading through a population, even if that is not the intention. Framing herd immunity as a deliberate strategy, as those television interviews seemed to do, sounded more sinister. There was a public perception that the government planned to let the virus sweep through the country without doing much to stop it.

That is not something, I believe, that anyone on SAGE could have meaningfully advocated. You only need a pen and the back of an envelope to clock the grim statistics of taking it all in one go: if herd immunity requires 60 per cent of people to become infected and one per cent of people die, this translates into roughly 40 million out of 66 million catching the disease – and about 400,000 of them dying. There would be added deaths among people unable to get treatment for other life-threatening diseases or emergencies, because hospital wards would be overrun with Covid-19 patients.

Patrick is, I believe, mortified at what happened. His defence is that he said the wrong thing and I am sure he regrets using the phrase 'herd immunity'. Any attempt to assign logic or meaning to what was going on also underestimates the unbelievable chaos of that period, when everyone was stretched beyond their limits.

It was a very intense and nervy period. People were absolutely shattered: working 18 hours a day; suddenly thrust into a political maelstrom and in front of TV cameras when they are not used to constant exposure; frightened they are going to get everything wrong and hundreds of thousands of people are going to die. Under that stress, people end up blurting out things they have not thought through. I don't believe there was any conspiracy inside government to kill people off; from what I saw, there was no plan.

It is true that SAGE thought that shutting down society would be really hard on people, especially on the poor, the vulnerable and the marginalised. That has proven to be true, with exactly those groups, and the young, suffering terrible hardship. Shuttering a nation would never be a step to be taken lightly. But acknowledging the difficulties with these unprecedented measures did not mean that drastic measures could never be on the table, especially when countries like Italy were taking robust action. The data in early March showed we were running out of options. Many of us wish we had been blunter and clearer with our comments, and that SAGE minutes had more fully reflected the long and agonising discussions on NPIs that took place.

Trying to pursue herd immunity as the virus thundered towards us would have been a dangerous gamble. The vulnerable would have required protecting and, while we knew back in February 2020 that the old were at higher risk of severe illness than the young, we would not have known who else to protect. Was it just the old? What about the young, patients on chemotherapy, people with immune disorders, people who have had transplants, pregnant women? The idea that you could hermetically seal off probably 20 per cent of society, maybe even more, and say, 'We're going to put you in a box for a few months, maybe a year,' was not feasible, practical, desirable or ethical.

Pursuing a fast 'herd immunity by natural infection' strategy would not have been 'following the science', as was so often claimed at that time, but doing the opposite. It went against the science. We have very little herd immunity to circulating coronaviruses that cause the common cold, which is why we are repeatedly infected. We have no idea if there is any long-lasting immunity to the related coronaviruses SARS-CoV-1 and Middle East respiratory virus. Back then, because of our lack of immunological knowledge, we could not have assumed herd immunity by natural infection was even viable for Covid-19, let alone safe. It is not a twenty-first-century public health plan. The idea of pursuing such an idea three months into a new disease beggared belief.

As far as I was concerned, the way forward in late-February was: to accept elimination was not possible (because of early, widespread seeding); reduce transmission; get R below 1; flatten the peak; stay within NHS limits; buy time to put measures like testing, tracing and isolation in place; increase NHS capacity; and to develop drugs and vaccines.

If Patrick had come to SAGE and said, 'Our plan is to take it on the chin and go for herd immunity by natural infection,' I would have resigned.

5

*If the plan is chicken pox parties, we're fucked**

10 MARCH 2020

Known global cases: 113,702
Global deaths: 4,012
UK cases: 373; UK deaths: 6

WHILE MANY OF US were sceptical about China-style lockdowns, Steven Riley had a different take. 'I thought what they did in Wuhan was brilliant,' he says. 'They didn't know it would work. Nobody did. But China taking the decision to throw everything at it was the only thing that gave the rest of the world a chance.'

Steven is a colleague of Neil's at Imperial College in London and a member of the SPI-M group of modellers. Like me, he had seen his February half-term family skiing holiday swallowed up by the Wuhan coronavirus as he built a mathematical model of how the virus might spread. He spent the day-long

---

* 'There was a clear division between the older, more senior people thinking, "Hang on, I thought this was the plan and there was no alternative" and the younger people thinking, "If the plan is chicken pox parties, we're fucked".'
Dominic Cummings, chief adviser to UK prime minister Boris Johnson.

107

train journey with his wife and three daughters, from London to Méribel in France, on his laptop writing code for his own model of how the outbreak would unfold in the UK, to which he could add data as it rolled in. He is quick to point out that he wasn't in *that* Méribel, the playground of the rich, but in a cheaper resort a bit further up the mountains, holidaying with other young families: 'People call it the Birmingham of the Alps but it's really nice,' he says.

The whole time, he was scrolling his phone for updates: 'There was one particular moment when I read about sustained human-to-human transmission. When I saw the virus was taking off in Iran and Italy, I knew it was going to be bad. I could see only two possible paths: either the UK was going to have loads of infections or it was going to have to do what China had done.' That night, in the Birmingham of the Alps, Steven got drunk for the first time in ten years.

On his return to the UK, his modelling stayed largely in the background until the second week of March 2020, when he became jittery at government inaction. On 9 March, he started putting together a paper for a meeting of the SPI-M modelling subgroup due to take place the next day. Steven explains: 'There was clearly a sense within government that there could be a fast way through this epidemic, that we could weather it by letting it pass through us quickly. The point of my note was to say "No".' He stayed up into the early hours to finish writing it; his wife, Michelle Heys, a clinical epidemiologist in the NHS, helped him to nail down its stark final paragraphs. Steven says he could not have written it without her.

Steven then agonised over whether to send it in. At 6.02am on 10 March he sent me an email headlined 'Managed acquisition immunity', with the note attached.

Hi Jeremy,
these are strange times and I am sorry to send you this out
of the blue. But I trust your judgement even though we don't
know each other that well…

I have been drafting this for nearly two weeks, hoping I
wouldn't have to send it. I have seen nothing that stops me
sending it.

As best you can, can you let me have some comments and
then answer two questions:

– will it help if I put this on record at UK gov
– would you do it if you were me

… I see it as totally justified on the precautionary principle.

Thanks in advance
Steven

The attached note explained why herd immunity would
not work and why containment was needed as quickly and
strongly as possible: because of how people were likely to
behave when faced with a serious pathogen.

The note drew on Steven's experience of studying a 2003
outbreak of SARS in Hong Kong. The initial surge of infections looked like the beginning of a pandemic but then the
outbreak mysteriously faded away. Steven and colleagues
had been trying to work out why. They eventually concluded
that the course of the epidemic changed because people
altered their behaviour in response to seeing residents of a
tower block being taken to quarantine facilities.

Similarly, Steven argued in the note, an epidemic could
not rip through the UK population quickly because people
would shut themselves away as infection rates rocketed and
intensive care units filled up, just as Hong Kong citizens
did. 'You're not going to carry on behaving as if the virus

isn't here if your local intensive care unit is full,' he says. If people preemptively changed their behaviour by locking themselves down before the virus had swept through the population, they would not acquire herd immunity. That would snatch away the only theoretical advantage of a fast epidemic, leaving behind mass casualties, a trashed health system and an epidemic that would still take a long time to run.

He wrote: 'The country would then have to either struggle on to the availability of a vaccine without a functioning health system or attempt the most stringent possible interventions to lower incidence back to containment levels. Over the same period of time, either of these scenarios would likely have far greater economic costs than would result from an immediate switch now to ongoing containment.'

To paraphrase his note: a herd immunity strategy, certainly one that aimed to get the epidemic over and done with quickly, would be the worst of all worlds. A fast epidemic would not achieve its sole objective, namely herd immunity, and the failure would come at enormous human and economic cost.

Steven had also read the report of an early WHO mission to China, leading him to conclude that it really was lockdown, not natural herd immunity, that was causing transmission in Wuhan to fall. By then, he noted, China's approach had been emulated by Hong Kong, Singapore, Japan, Vietnam and South Korea.* The falling infection rates in those countries, Steven wrote, were 'strong evidence with which to abandon mitigation [herd immunity] strategies, justified in any way by the possibility of a short epidemic. Governments need to devote the entirety of their attention and resources to creating

---

* A *Lancet* study published in March 2020 found that about 7 per cent of Wuhan citizens had antibodies to the virus, suggesting lockdown rather than natural herd immunity was cutting transmission.

viable ongoing solutions to the presence of this virus. We suggest that the first step is to adopt stringent fixed-term social distancing.' The UK going into lockdown, he argued, would provide a breathing space for ministers to work out what to do next.

But he was nervous about offering a contrarian viewpoint, which is why he had asked for my advice. China was reportedly going to extreme lengths to enforce its lockdowns, such as welding shut the doors to apartment blocks. I could understand his reticence to endorse the China way: I had recently been invited on to the Christiane Amanpour TV show in the US, which showed distressing footage of a woman who could not cross a police barrier to take her daughter for cancer therapy.

Steven says: 'I couldn't get that story about the doors being welded shut out of my mind. I don't even know if it was true. There was a narrative developing that China's lockdown succeeded because it was a communist country. But just because China looks different from us didn't mean we wouldn't be able to do it. I was worried about Michelle and the NHS in general. We'd had dinner with medic friends on 6 March and there was a real disconnect between what they were expecting and what we were expecting.'

His argument found a willing audience. John says: 'Steven brought this simple note to the table that said, "Look, enough is enough, this isn't working and we should go into lockdown." And that's what we all kind of felt. It was the government's job to set strategy and our role to find a way of making it work. But we just couldn't, not without hundreds of thousands of deaths. Every combination of measures that we modelled ended up with way more hospitalisations than the NHS could cope with. And we modelled everything but a full lockdown.'

There was vigorous discussion among modellers through the evening of 10 March and into the early hours of 11 March. John recalls: 'We were thinking, could we really go into lockdown and just wait for a vaccine? But Steven was basically right: it was better to fail from that position [lockdown] than letting the epidemic run.'

In the middle of the night, John and colleagues realised that intermittent lockdowns might offer a slower, less deadly middle road between an unexpurgated epidemic and an open-ended lockdown. It would more comfortably keep the epidemic within the limits of the NHS, ensuring, in theory at least, that everyone who needed treatment could get it.

Intermittent lockdowns would go on and off like a switch as needed, applied on top of milder restrictions when healthcare systems looked in danger of being overrun. The milder restrictions would slow the epidemic down like taking the foot off an accelerator; Wuhan-style lockdowns would act as an emergency brake when surveillance showed cases were dangerously on the rise.

Modellers at the London School of Hygiene and Tropical Medicine took the lead on finessing the model. The approach would see the epidemic running its course over 18 months, with perhaps around 100,000 deaths. That was massively higher than anyone wanted, but it halved the projected deaths from all the alternatives. Immunity via natural infection, if it existed, might slowly build up in the population, holding out a slim hope of the UK epidemic subsiding even if a vaccine never arrived. Some of the harms, known and unknown, of long-term lockdowns could be avoided.

It was still, technically, a managed herd immunity strategy but over a longer period of time that would leave fewer deaths in its wake. If that sounds callous, it is worth stepping back into the spring of 2020. To say there was uncertainty about how things would play out is an extreme understatement. A Covid-19 vaccine could not be guaranteed – ever. We did not know of any successful treatments or other cures. If we were going to be stuck with this virus for years, the UK needed a sustainable way of trying to keep infections low while keeping some of society running (especially schools). This was not 'taking it on the chin'.

'Intermittent lockdowns allowed us to get to herd immunity but without half a million deaths,' John says. 'You could also change strategy as you went along. If a vaccine came along, you could stay in lockdown until it could be rolled out.' Even so, adopting it was still a decision for government, not SAGE.

❋ ❋ ❋

On Wednesday 11 March 2020, the World Health Organization declared the coronavirus outbreak a pandemic. Classing an outbreak as a pandemic just means the outbreak has spread, or has the capacity to spread, everywhere on earth. SARS-CoV-2 had reached every continent bar Antarctica; there were now more than 118,000 cases globally and nearly 4,300 deaths. It did not materially change anything, other than to formally recognise what we already knew: SARS-CoV-2 was infecting the world.

John, meanwhile, had been cleaning up and plugging in the sentinel surveillance data he'd been sent a few days earlier by Public Health England (PHE). These were cases that had come to light via a network of GP surgeries testing randomly for the virus and hospitals testing patients admitted with severe pneumonia. Modellers had been pushing for sentinel testing and surveillance for weeks. The new data would allow a more accurate guesstimate on how many cases the UK was harbouring, and how the epidemic was progressing. At the SAGE meeting on 10 March, advisers had been told there were 5,000 to 10,000 cases in the UK in total.

When John fed the PHE data into the models to calculate how the epidemic was playing out in the UK, the results looked off – and not in a good way: 'We worked out from scaling up the PHE data that the epidemic was growing by anything from a few hundred to 5,000 new infections a day. Our central estimate was 1,500–2,000 a day, doubling every five to six days.' Working backwards meant that the true number of infected people in the UK was closer to 30,000, a far cry from the 5,000–10,000 mentioned at SAGE.

John had promised to visit a friend to watch the Champions League football match between Liverpool and Atlético Madrid on 11 March but skipped it to help colleagues Mark Jit and Thibaut Jombart sort the discrepancy out. They could not make it go away. They approached Graham Medley, who chairs SPI-M and is also at the London School of Hygiene and Tropical Medicine. Graham was himself so alarmed at the results that he hastily arranged for PHE to triple-check it using their own models.

On 12 March, PHE confirmed their fears: the UK was nursing an epidemic that was adding a ballpark figure of 800 new infections a day and doubling every three to four days. 'On the face of it, 800 a day sounded less bad than 1,500,' John says, 'but because it was doubling more quickly, it was actually worse news.' It seems hard to believe now but, on that same day, it was announced that community testing for Covid-19 was to be dropped. Testing would only take place in hospitals. I did not know this was coming and no convincing reason was given.

That night, I sent an email to Neil and John:

Date: Thursday, 12 March 2020 at 21:05

To: John Edmunds, Neil Ferguson

Subject: UKG and COVID

Are you both comfortable with the plans UKG [UK government] have got in place, the pace of actions and the changes they are making?

Neil feared the modelling scenarios were still being viewed, wrongly, as extremely unlikely.

John sent a one-line reply: 'NO I AM NOT'.

✳ ✳ ✳

The next SAGE meeting was held, aptly, on Friday 13 March 2020. It opened with the ominous news that the UK was further along its epidemic than anyone realised. The atmosphere of apprehension was deepened by the nature of the venue: not the expansive basement we had become used to but a tiny, airless seventh-floor room in a different building on Victoria Street. It was packed, with everyone on top of each other. I was wedged between Steve Powis, from the NHS, and Charlotte Watts, an epidemiologist at the London School of Hygiene and Tropical Medicine and chief scientific adviser to the Department for International Development. I remember thinking it would be the perfect place for an infectious disease to spread.

In that SAGE meeting, two important datasets were about to collide for the first time: infection numbers and NHS capacity. For Neil, the UK epidemic was speeding into focus with frightening clarity: 'In that week running up to the SAGE meeting on 13 March, we were starting to get more data through on how quickly things were moving in the UK. I think that changed views within government and in Patrick Vallance and Chris Whitty's minds; they became more convinced that the scenarios we had been modelling would happen. Reality was dawning on people.' The reasonable worst-case scenarios were being seen anew as the most likely scenarios, as they should have been from the beginning.

On NHS capacity, I remember Steve Powis pulling out a file which showed bed occupancy and the number of ventilators available around the country. The take-home message was: if the modelling of Neil and John and Steven Riley and others came to pass, using the improved surveillance data that was coming in, then the NHS would be in dire peril. We would go the way of Italy. That was the first time, on Friday 13 March 2020, we had sight of the data signposting that catastrophic scenario: that the NHS was about to collapse.

But few would have guessed it from the minutes.* When I later read them, I genuinely wondered how I could have been at the same table. Minutes in large organisations, and particularly government departments, can be very anodyne, providing wiggle room for interpretation afterwards. In any meeting like that, the desire to get a clear message across must be weighed against the fear of instilling panic. But the horror unfolding in Italy meant that panic was called for.

And yet the SAGE minutes for Friday 13 March began: 'Owing to a 5–7 day lag in data provision for modelling, SAGE now believes there are more cases in the UK than SAGE previously expected at this point, and we may therefore be further ahead on the epidemic curve, but the UK remains on broadly the same epidemic trajectory and time to peak.'

---

* The minutes improved hugely from Easter onwards, and by autumn there were no such ambiguities. I am grateful to the SAGE secretariat, which has worked extremely hard throughout.

That undersold the magnitude of what was coming our way – and did not emphasise that it would hit sooner than had been assumed. I had left that very same SAGE meeting on Friday 13 March convinced that Wellcome's offices and public spaces should be closed immediately. A statement was posted on our website that day, saying the shutters would go up on Monday 16 March until further notice. Privately, I was contemplating whether our London HQ could house make-shift facilities if neighbouring University College Hospital ran out of space.

There was no need to rush the introduction of NPIs, the minutes continued reassuringly; any closures or restrictions would be hard to sustain. There would be 'minor gains' from enacting these early. Banning sporting events and large gatherings would have negligible impact, the minutes recorded, with greater risk coming from small, informal, close gatherings; good news for those involved with the Cheltenham Gold Cup, a horse-racing festival due to take place that weekend. In truth, both sporting events and large gatherings should have been stopped earlier. But closing pubs, bars and restaurants, it was advised, would have greater impact on transmission.

The key takeaway for many of us on that Friday, that the NHS was on the brink of disaster, was buried further down: 'There is a risk that current proposed measures (individual and household isolation and social distancing) will not reduce [NHS] demand enough.' Almost as an aside, the minutes noted that community testing was being dropped that day.

Late into the evening on Saturday 14 March, I bashed out a hurried email to Patrick and Chris, marking it 'in confidence':

I know how desperately hard this is, the hours being worked under enormous stress by everyone in the system and a huge amount being done – trying to be constructive. Thought long and hard whether to send.

Are you content that these minutes convey:

The need for urgency that was palpable at the meeting

The speed that this is unfolding

We are further ahead in the epidemic – not 'we may be'

The framing of the modelling, and the behavioural science comes with a lot of uncertainties and caveats

Impatience that the diagnostic testing lags behind and that there are 'plans' to ramp up to 1000tests/week at some point?

Not sure when the decision to stop testing in the community was made – is that right, no more testing of community non-hospitalised cases?

The significant lag between any decisions and impact, such a time lag in a fast-moving epidemic is concerning

The need for social distancing interventions to be implemented as soon as policy could be written and communicated – very soon

Need for comprehensive suite of social distancing interventions

Increase in capacity in the NHS – an operational issue but clearly a critical one

In next 24 hours

* Act early and decisively

* Open access to all the evidence being used within UKG [UK government]

* Shift in policy on social distancing with immediate effect and across all – working from home whenever possible, work places, mass gatherings, religious meetings, restaurants/bars/ cinemas, public transport, advice to shops, limit number of people in shops and other places – etc,

* Home quarantine for suspected cases and family for 14 days

* 'Shielding' of vulnerable populations

* Economic support for businesses, self-employed etc – Fair and equity

* If possible keep schools open until Easter (2 weeks) to avoid staffing issues within NHS – but within schools actions such as pushing hand washing, no assemblies, break up classes into smaller units, no gatherings etc etc

* Massive increase capacity in the NHS

* Massively increased diagnostic capacity

* Support through G7 for R&D and Manufacturing of Diagnostics, Therapeutics and Vaccines

* Clear lines of decision making and control – may not be a time to keep a consensus if that means delaying inevitable decisions

* Increase the capacity, demands and expectations on DHSC, PHE, NHS and single line of decision making...

I believe these changes needed in the next 24 hours – doubling time now 2.5–3 days

I hit 'send'.

Separately, I also told Patrick and Chris that Wellcome was closing. It was intended as a friendly heads-up in case someone thought to ask the obvious question: what did Wellcome know about this virus that the UK government did not?

* * *

It was not just scientists nursing a sense of foreboding. In late February and early March, Dominic Cummings had begun to worry about the UK's pandemic response: 'There was no proper coordination in my opinion between SAGE, the Department of Health, the NHS and the Cabinet Office. Things were clearly being garbled. Everyone thought lots of things were different people's responsibilities. That's why I asked Ben Warner to start attending SAGE.'

Cummings is the notorious figure behind the Vote Leave campaign, which took the UK out of the European Union. I had not met him before the coronavirus crisis and only knew of him by reputation, as a rather intimidating political operator but interested in science. While I had no time for his views on Brexit, I felt that during this crisis he was a force for good inside government. In meetings at Number 10 and elsewhere, he was always curious, asked the right probing questions of the science and had the capacity to spot the difference between good-quality evidence and bogus science. He listened intently and seemed to be one of the few people who could make things happen at speed across government.

Ben Warner is a data scientist who trained at University College London and worked with Cummings at Vote Leave. During February and March 2020, Warner frequently attended SAGE meetings. Cummings also called upon the expertise of Marc Warner, Ben's brother and also a data scientist, who founded a company called Faculty. Marc had also been involved with Vote Leave and had recently been drafted in to work with NHS Digital.

Cummings offers his own account of what happened in this important period, which echoes but also adds to the seven hours of evidence he gave to UK MPs on 26 May 2021. Ben Warner was at that fateful SAGE meeting on Friday 13 March 2020 and clearly picked up the extreme anxiety in the room. His message back to Cummings that night was that there had been a horrible miscalculation: data now indicated the NHS would collapse long before the epidemic peaked, possibly within a month. Cummings recalls: 'On that Friday night, Ben Warner said to said to me and Imran [Imran Shafi, Boris Johnson's private secretary], "I think this herd immunity plan is going to be a catastrophe. The NHS is going to be destroyed. We should try to lock everything down as fast as we possibly can."' That was my view, and I am sure most people on SAGE agreed.

Cummings was also courting the views of three scientists beyond SAGE, to whom he was occasionally sending SAGE papers: Venki Ramakrishnan, president of the Royal Society and a chemistry Nobel laureate; Demis Hassabis; and Timothy Gowers, the British mathematician and Fields medallist. I saw both Demis and Venki at the odd SAGE meeting but not Timothy.

Timothy told Cummings in a series of emails that, in his view, the best strategy was to go in hard and early on interventions like lockdowns, because of exponential growth in case numbers. Timothy explains the reasoning he gave to Cummings: 'I felt very strongly at the time that a herd immunity strategy was wrong – a simple back-of-the-envelope calculation made it clear that in order to implement it, either hospitals would have to be massively overwhelmed or the strategy would take years, and depend on reinfection not being possible ... Given that a herd immunity strategy couldn't possibly work, lockdown was inevitable, and that given that lockdown was inevitable, it was madness not to start immediately.' All it needed, Timothy says, was an understanding of basic mathematics.

Cummings claims he was also being contacted by other people he knew, such as Patrick Collison, the Irish billion-aire founder of online payments platform Stripe, who were convinced the UK was heading for disaster and needed to change course.

Ben Warner's SOS from the SAGE meeting on Friday 13 March prompted Cummings to arrange a flurry of meetings in Downing Street on Saturday 14 and Sunday 15 March, to tell Johnson of the need to take action.

Cummings claims that, as well as a 9am official meeting in the Cabinet Room on Saturday morning that has been widely reported, a second meeting took place at around 11am on Saturday morning in the PM's office. The attendees were Cummings; Ben Warner and Marc Warner; Boris Johnson; Imran Shafi; advisers Lee Cain and Cleo Watson; and Laura Pimpin, the chief epidemiologist at Babylon Health, a digital healthcare company. Health secretary Matt Hancock wanted to join, but Cummings says he shut the door in his face (Cummings is scathing of Hancock's handling of the crisis and said he wanted him sacked).

Cummings says: 'I brought Laura in because we had nobody in Number 10 who seemed to know what a disease or a virus was. I knew her, and asked Babylon to lend her, which they did. Laura was one of the people shouting at me that week that I needed to stop this somehow. I got Ben Warner and Marc Warner to go through the actual data and we basically said to the PM, "This whole wave is going to peak much faster than [June] and is going to destroy the NHS in the next month. A lot of people in the Cabinet Office and Department of Health haven't clocked the difference between time to peak and time to NHS collapse, which is an extremely big and important difference, and unless you change tack shortly we're going to kill half a million people."' Cummings told Johnson there was not even a plan to bury all the dead: 'In the chaos the whole grip of government might collapse with all sorts of other terrible consequences.'

Afterwards, Cummings said he rang Patrick and told him the government needed a Plan B, because 'it was clear parts of the system didn't understand the consequences of Plan A, that DHSC [Department of Health and Social Care] and the Cabinet seemed to be dangerously uncoordinated and many had not understood the implications of the graphs.' Cummings recalls: 'Patrick said, "I agree, it's clear the policy machine is broken somewhere and I don't understand where. We've got to try to move everything faster."'

Cummings asked Patrick to come to Downing Street on Sunday, to present Plan B to Johnson. The new plan, a move to suppression, was yet to be decided.

❋ ❋ ❋

Even if the minutes were hazy, I believe that Patrick and Chris took a clear message into Number 10 after that Friday 13 March SAGE meeting: measures had to start immediately. Meanwhile, my email to Patrick and Chris on Saturday 14 March 2020 tried to capture very explicitly what was hampering the UK's ability to respond.

First, the state of public health at the time a country enters a crisis is crucial. In February, Public Health England could cope with perhaps five coronavirus cases per week. It was the kind of testing capacity you might expect in a low-income country: you cannot invent resources that are not there, and therefore, if a crisis hits, you have to ration them.

Neither can you turn on capacity when you need it because everyone is chasing the same items. This virus was on every continent: there was a shortage of absolutely everything, from the enzymes needed for the tests, to the tests themselves. We were hearing outrageous stories of countries outbidding each other in airport hangars, to poach PPE supplies already contractually promised elsewhere.

So, faced with a capacity of five cases a week, where would that testing bring the most benefit? It had to be in hospital. That renders the tip of the iceberg visible. But it meant dropping community testing (Cummings claims it was dropped as part of the herd immunity plan).

Embarrassingly, around the time of that decision on 12 March, the WHO was urging countries to 'test, test, test'. I remember Jenny Harries, England's deputy chief medical officer, saying publicly that the UK did not need to follow the WHO's advice because it did not apply to high-income countries. It was a dreadful thing to say. There was no public acknowledgement that abandoning community testing was a decision based not on public health or science considerations but on a lack of testing capacity. It meant we were flying blind when it came to transmission outside of hospitals, in the community and in care homes.

The idosyncratic British approach baffled observers at the WHO, including Maria Van Kerkhove, in the Health Emergencies Programme and a key figure in the agency's Covid-19 response. Maria recalls: 'The attitude was, "Don't worry, that's China, that's not here. That's Lombardy, that's not here. We've got this." I heard many people on UK media in the beginning say, "No, that won't happen here, we have a very strong health system that will deal with it, nothing to see here." Many other countries did the same thing. It was hubris.'

The fact that the UK did not have eyes on the virus had serious consequences: the UK could not see the epidemic as it truly was, making it harder to calculate how it was developing. As John Edmunds says: 'The data was terrible and we had poor situational awareness.' Second, a crisis cries out for clear lines of command and control. We were navigating a very fragmented set of decision-making processes, and there was uncertainty about who answered to whom. Every government department has a chief scientist who reports to Patrick. Patrick and Chris are peers, and they both have a complicated relationship with NHS England, led by Simon Stevens. Then there's the Department of Health and Social Care led by a Cabinet minister, Matt Hancock, who has only partial control over what Simon Stevens does. On top of that is Public Health England, plus the Home Office, Foreign and Commonwealth Office, Department for Education and others. Devolution adds further complexity: Scotland, Wales and Northern Ireland do things slightly differently.

Hearing now about the turmoil inside Number 10 that weekend adds weight to what I and many others felt at the time: there was huge uncertainty about who was ultimately taking responsibility for the pandemic response. Boris Johnson as prime minister seemed more like an old-fashioned chairman than a chief executive and was being advised by Dominic Cummings and other figures in Number 10. It was unclear who was pulling the strings and who had the authority to ask, let alone compel, others to act.

Cummings shares the view that general confusion reigned in that period: 'Nothing worked. The preparations were a farce, the plan was a catastrophe and had to be abandoned, and the management of many crucial things was a disaster.'

And his boss had not been paying attention. Cummings adds: 'The PM spent most of February dealing with a combination of divorce, his current girlfriend wanting to make announcements about their relationship, an ex-girlfriend running around the media, financial problems exacerbated by the flat renovation, his book on Shakespeare, and other nonsense, because obviously he never took the whole thing seriously.'

The absence of leadership became even more apparent when Johnson became ill with coronavirus towards the end of March and Dominic Raab, the foreign secretary, took over.

I felt we were missing a figure to pull it all together, like Jeremy Heywood, the late cabinet secretary and head of the civil service, who I had met during the Ebola crisis. That is what the Cabinet Office is there for: to make sure government works as a whole, especially in a crisis. Jeremy's successor, Mark Sedwill, seemed, to me, absent in that role. He ended up leaving government in difficult circumstances in September 2020. His departure had been ascribed to a clash of opinions over Brexit, the UK's departure from the European Union, the other cataclysmic event then preoccupying ministerial minds. I also wondered at the apparent absence of Michael Gove, minister for the Cabinet Office.

The Joint Biosecurity Centre, set up in May 2020 and modelled on the Joint Terrorism Analysis Centre based in MI5, has gone a long way to becoming a nerve centre. It pulls in information from SAGE and from other sources, such as mobile phone data, which can help to model behaviour changes and adherence to lockdowns. It has been excellent at turning huge amounts of data into usable information that can feed into policy and has genuinely transformed the UK pandemic response for the better. Something like this needs to be running from day 1 of week 1, not day 4 of week 20.

Third, there is a time lag between advice being given and that advice being acted on, or operationalised. It takes time to pull levers, and for the impact of the pulling to be felt. That is, if pulling a lever had an impact at all. I felt strongly that the levers being pulled sometimes had nothing on the end of them.

Time lags are a consequence, in part, of piecemeal decision-making. There is an understandable desire for consensus as critical decisions are being made. Then, that advice must be translated into action. Each step builds in a delay. But time is the one thing you do not have in a fast-moving epidemic. Delays matter when an epidemic is doubling every three days.

For one thing, you are always viewing data in the rear-view mirror. The number of cases, hospitalisations and deaths today reveals the state of the epidemic days or weeks ago, not the state of the epidemic today. Today's data reflects the past.

That can be hard to grasp but must be factored into decision-making. If today's data tells you there were 1,000 cases three days ago, then in reality there are at least 2,000 today – and in the next doubling time you'll have 4,000 cases. Every delay means more infections, which inevitably means more hospitalisations and more deaths. Before you know it, you have lost control. On Saturday 14 March, as I wrote in the email, I felt action was needed within 24 hours: basically lockdown, plus all the other measures that had been modelled, like Italy and other European countries had done.

That period reminded me powerfully of what Carter Mecher had said in late January, in the emails with Richard Hatchett and other US figures predicting we would not be able to outrun this one. We needed to keep asking ourselves this: in two weeks or a month from now, what would we wish we had done today?

Cummings knows now what should have happened: 'In retrospect, it's obvious that if we locked down a week earlier that would have been better; two weeks earlier would have been better still ... It's just unarguable from my perspective that everything we did should have happened earlier. Fewer people would have died, lockdown would have been shorter

127

and we would have had less economic destruction.' He believes that tens of thousands, even hundreds of thousands, more people would have died if no action had been taken for a fortnight, which he claims could 'easily have happened given the then current plans'.

At his appearance before MPs, Cummings apologised for the fact that he and others had let the country down and that tens of thousands of people died who did not need to die. That people died needlessly is, alas, unarguable from any insider's perspective.

� ✳ ✳ ✳

Cummings denies conceiving or pushing a herd immunity strategy at Number 10, saying he believed it came from SAGE: 'I kept asking repeatedly why we couldn't do what Singapore were doing, because Singapore is a very well-run country and had been through SARS and MERS. We were told repeatedly that SAGE thought there was no alternative to herd immunity because any kind of [lockdown] strategy like China or Taiwan or Singapore wouldn't work, would only create a second, uncontainable peak in the winter when the NHS was overstretched and there wouldn't be any vaccines for at least a year. I would swear to that on a stack of Bibles and so would everyone else in Number 10 including the prime minister, and for once he wouldn't be lying.'[*]

Michael Parker, an ethicist at Oxford University who was not on SAGE at the time but was invited to join soon after, perhaps because of the herd immunity controversy, was also wondering why the UK was refusing to lift its gaze east: 'The

---

[*] Cummings's opinions on controversial scientific issues have raised eyebrows. In a 2014 blog on 'designer babies', he argued that the NHS should cover the cost of embryo selection of high IQ babies, should such technology become available.

really important question for me is, why didn't we just look at South East Asia, at China, at South Korea and the other countries who were leaping into action? It was clear what they were doing was having an impact. The huge mistake was thinking that, because there are important cultural and political differences, nothing could be learnt from countries or groups of people. That is a kind of racism. It meant we failed to make the most of the time we had, and we paid the price.'

I do not buy into the idea that Cummings was a herd immunity enthusiast. Neither does Timothy Gowers: 'The narrative that [Cummings] was callous about human life is wrong. My reading of the situation is he was trying to follow what he thought was the best scientific advice at the time.'

Cummings, who caught Covid-19, is still upset at being framed as its architect: '[Those accusations were] made by a combination of people inside the system who hated me or wanted rid of me, who were briefing, "Cummings has come up with this." Then you had the insane Remainer social media networks going, "Oh my god, the evil Cummings is now going to try and kill everyone!"'

Cummings' belief that the government was being advised by SAGE to chase herd immunity was underscored, he says, by the conversations in Number 10 comparing the strategy to chicken pox parties. On 12 March 2020, Ben Warner asked Number 10 officials to stop using the analogy, pointing out that chicken pox was not going to kill half a million people. That remark, Cummings recalls, stunned those present: 'There was a clear division between the older, more senior people thinking, "Hang on, I thought this was the plan and there was no alternative," and the younger people thinking, "If the plan is chicken pox parties, we're fucked."'

This analogy would never have come from SAGE.

Cummings emphasises that Patrick Vallance and Chris Whitty were always scrupulous in their presentation of SAGE discussions: 'They were always careful to say, "This is not policy advice", and I was careful to say, "We understand, you're not telling us what policy should be, that's our job. But what you are saying very explicitly is the Chinese plan will fail, the Singapore plan will fail, the Taiwan plan will fail and everyone's basically going to have to do herd immunity," right?' I do not believe that Chris and Patrick, or SAGE, would ever have knowingly agreed to that.

Cummings now believes that both sides became trapped 'in a kind of mental, psychological or epistemological loop. People in SAGE were thinking, (A) there's no political appetite for lockdown because the PM doesn't really believe in it, (B) the public won't accept lockdown anyway because the behavioural science says so, and therefore (C) that encourages the idea that we are just going to go for herd immunity because we can't do suppression. That's what seems to me to be going on.'

Cummings says he wishes he had interrogated the behavioural science assumptions more carefully: 'That is one of the things that I blame myself for. A lot of people started babbling theories about behaviour and communications [about why the UK could not lock down]. I spent a lot of time looking at this in the context of the Brexit referendum and I knew that a lot of smart people have completely bonkers ideas about it ... Both Ben Warner and I said we did not believe this idea that the public won't accept lockdowns, or won't accept a test and trace system. You could see the TV pictures of Lombardy. We were getting messages from our own friends and family saying, "What is going on down there, when are you going to lock down?"'

I do not believe that behavioural scientists on SAGE ever claimed that the public would not accept lockdowns. The scientists themselves have rejected Cummings' assertions and point out that it was not their role to suggest interventions, only to advise on how people should be encouraged to adhere to whatever interventions that ministers chose. And I was told that ministers were universally opposed to even household isolation. We understood that people would comply with measures if the rationale was explained, the reasons were transparent, they were applied consistently, and they were not disadvantaged by complying. It is still the case that the government must own the strategy it pursued, rather than hide behind the scientists. Cummings says he thought these ideas originated on SPI-B or SAGE, but I dispute this. It should be noted that the UK government does have its own Behavioural Insights team and David Halpern (head of that team) gave the first interview mentioning herd immunity.

This bitterly contested issue – over where the science that informed the UK pandemic response came from – highlights the lack of people inside Number 10 with the technical expertise to challenge poor science.

※ ※ ※

On Monday 16 March 2020, I and other SAGE advisers found ourselves back in the cavernous basement meeting room at 10 Victoria Street. The view in the rear-view mirror was changing alarmingly. At the meeting, and recorded in the minutes, we heard that there could be as many as 10,000 cases in London alone. The doubling time was estimated at five to six days. That was longer than I had guessed – but these were still staggering figures.

Still, we had clear evidence that the lockdowns in China and other countries were bending the curve the right way. We were being chastened daily by the tales from critical care units in Italy; on 15 March, cases in Italy had risen to nearly 25,000, with more than 1,800 deaths. It was surely time for action. If we needed yet another compelling reason to act, 'Report 9' fitted the bill.

This paper was a pivotal piece of epidemiological modelling led by Neil's team. The team had modelled how the epidemic might progress if left to its own devices. If no preventive measures were taken, and if people did not change behaviour of their own accord – an 'unmitigated' epidemic – Neil's team calculated that around 80 per cent of the population would become infected. With an overall infection fatality rate of 0.9 per cent, 510,000 people would die in the UK and more than 2 million in the US. For comparison, there were an estimated 384,000 deaths among British forces in the Second World War.

The modelling also painted a grim picture of how such an epidemic curve would play out in real life: intensive care beds running out by early April; at the peak, 30 patients competing for each bed, meaning 29 of them turned away, probably to die.

Even the mitigating measures discussed at SAGE until that point – isolation of known cases, household quarantining, shielding the over-70s – would be unable to keep hospital capacity from being overwhelmed. It would still lead to around 250,000 deaths. Suppression – bringing the epidemic down to manageable levels – would take all those measures plus social distancing of the entire population (like a full lockdown, except people are allowed to go to work).

This was the point that Steven Riley had been pushing, in raising the prospect of a China-style lockdown on the basis of the precautionary principle in his simple modelling note to SPI-M on 10 March. The strategy needed to switch immediately from mitigation to suppression – to try as hard as possible to stop the virus from circulating.

✻ ✻ ✻

After that 16 March SAGE meeting, held in the early afternoon, I actually felt optimistic that the UK was about to correct course. At just after 4pm, I sent a lengthy email to my colleagues at Wellcome:

South Korea, Hong Kong, Singapore have taken a fairly uniform approach [i.e. lockdown] and have been able to either reduce the peak, prevent community transmission or change the epidemic curve.

This has been very impressive and lessons should be learnt from what these countries have done.

The epicentre for this pandemic is very clearly now in Europe.

Continental Europe has taken a fairly uniform approach. The UK has (as of 15 March 2020) taken a different approach, that must and will change.

I anticipate seeing a major shift in strategy today [16 March 2020] which should be clear at the Press Conference from the PM today.

I threw in some good news: the first safety trials of a CEPI-funded coronavirus vaccine were due to start, at the US biotech company Moderna. I also wanted to mark, for my colleagues, the historic moment that a pandemic forced a retreat from our offices into our homes:

Over the coming weeks & months we will all be tired at times, fearful, we will make mistakes. These are very tough times. We will be short tempered & grumpy! But we will get through it and the togetherness, solidarity and support for each other is what we will remember. We are living through as history is made, events which will be discussed in 100 years time, as 1918 is discussed today.

That evening, I expected to hear that the shutters were going down everywhere in the UK, as we had done at Wellcome. Instead, when Boris Johnson appeared on TV, he asked people to work from home, to stop non-essential travel and avoid pubs, bars, restaurants and mass gatherings. Venues could remain open. The measures were being advised rather than mandated, and the PM, a self-confessed libertarian, made clear his reluctance to instigate them.

I was shocked: rather than taking a tough decision, the PM ducked it. Johnson, in fact, did exactly what SAGE had cautioned against at the 25 February meeting. Social distancing measures should be mandatory, not optional. A prime minister cannot ask people to lock down if they feel like it. No countries in South East Asia had done it this way, for good reason: that is not the way these sorts of public health measures work.

It is a fair criticism that the minutes from SAGE meetings do not explicitly show advisers calling for stronger action. I regret that SAGE was not blunter in that regard. We should have been, especially during that key weekend between Friday 13 and Monday 16 March; my Saturday email on 14 March was a late-night attempt to lay out the argument much more plainly and directly to Patrick and Chris that action, namely lockdown, was needed within 24 hours.

Still, there we were, on Monday 16 March 2020, with a half-measure that pleased neither the politicians nor the scientists: a voluntary semi-lockdown.

6

It's taken an emotional toll on everyone[*]

16 MARCH 2020

Known global cases: 167,515
Global deaths: 6,606
UK cases: 1,395; UK deaths: 35

DECIDING TO CLOSE AN ECONOMY is unbelievably tough. Other than during wars, Western economies had never had a lockdown since the Middle Ages, to my knowledge; this is just not something governments do. But the horror stories coming from Italy, a rich country just a two-hour flight from the UK where the health system was imploding, should have been evidence enough. With Spain not far behind, and France on a similar trajectory, it was denying reality to think we would be spared.

Yet the UK was suffering its own long-standing malady: the arrogance of exceptionalism. The UK is joined by other countries, including India and Brazil, in this failing. India

---

[*] 'It's taken an emotional toll on everyone.'
Neil Ferguson, Imperial College London.

declared victory against Covid-19 in February 2021, even passing a resolution congratulating Prime Minister Modi and his party, the BJP. Two months later, the country was engulfed by a truly apocalyptic second wave, thanks in part to the B.1.617 variants, which, at the time of writing is becoming the dominant strain globally.

The middle of March 2020 was a critical time period in the failure of the UK response. Frankly, I was amazed that the government had not moved more definitively. By this time, Wellcome, along with many organisations, had locked its doors – after a month of contingency planning.

With its lack of panic, the UK looked like an international outlier. Ministers, as well as Patrick and Chris, said the right measures would be taken at the right time. The belief was that people would only be able to comply with stringent social distancing measures for a limited period of time before 'behavioural fatigue' set in – and it would be dangerous if people threw in the towel just before the epidemic peaked.

Behavioural fatigue seems to have been a peripheral idea promoted beyond any merit or evidence. Behavioural scientists on SAGE had acknowledged that people might struggle to comply with restrictions, but had also, importantly, cautioned this was an intuitive observation, not one based on evidence. Besides, the danger was escalating and options were running out.

On 16 March 2020, nearly 700 psychologists and behavioural researchers released an open letter to the government asking for the relevant evidence on behavioural fatigue to be disclosed or, if there was no evidence, to change tack. They were 'not convinced that enough is known about "behavioural fatigue" or to what extent these insights apply to the current exceptional circumstances. Such evidence is necessary if we are to base a high-risk public health strategy on it...'

It was a constructive intervention. So, by 16 March, the judgement from outbreak veterans, epidemiological modellers and the UK's behavioural science community had reached a consensus: act now.

* * *

SAGE met again on Wednesday 18 March, a day on which 999 fresh coronavirus cases were reported across the UK. I sat between Demis Hassabis and Ian Diamond, the brilliant chief statistician at the Office for National Statistics. There were around a dozen advisers in the room, and as many others dialling in, plus a handful of SAGE administrative staff.

We were facing a terrible situation: the UK was estimated to be between two and four weeks behind Italy on its epidemic curve. That forecast was tallying with data from the NHS suggesting intensive care capacity would run out in London by early April. But we would not know for another three weeks whether the voluntary measures that the PM had urged on the public just two days earlier would head off disaster.

As London was ahead of other regions in its number of infections, with beds filling up fast, a separate COBR meeting, at which Cummings was present, discussed locking the capital down. The prospect of quarantining London elicited mixed feelings: some worried that urbanites would flee to second homes, seeding the virus in regions with fewer hospital beds. That had happened across the Channel: the French countryside was fizzing with discontent at the influx of potentially infected Parisians.

Number 10 also feared that a London lockdown would cause the stock market to crash. On 12 March 2020, the FTSE 100 index had seen the biggest one-day fall since Black Monday in 1987, dwarfing the loss of confidence caused by the 2008 financial crisis. The idea of quarantining the capital was abandoned: more than half the UK cases were already outside London anyway, having been strewn across the country by travellers returning from Europe.

The modelling, reprising the messages from the SAGE meetings on 13 and 16 March, showed that, to avert the horrendous tally of deaths coming our way, the country needed to do more than simply getting the vulnerable to shield, the infected to quarantine and affected households to isolate. A modelling paper by Nick Davies, one of John's colleagues, suggested that a nationwide shutting of schools and universities would buy some, though not much, respite. 'Even with school closure, the UK is likely to experience a large epidemic which will result in overwhelming demand for health services,' the paper concluded. Still, it would cut deaths by about 9 per cent.

Demis was doing some back-of-the-envelope maths using the numbers that he was hearing. It largely coincided with Neil and John's modelling showing that deaths would run into the hundreds of thousands. Startled, Demis cited the same concern that Steven Riley had raised with me: 'What about the precautionary principle?' If all the modelling was even partially accurate, and we were about to become the next Italy, the only intervention we had left available was to close down the economy. That meant shutting everything.

SAGE advised that schools should be closed as soon as possible, except possibly for the children of key workers; pubs, restaurants, other hospitality and leisure should shut, along with indoor workplaces. Any interventions should happen sooner rather than later, we advised once again. Strikingly, a YouGov poll showed that 16 per cent of school pupils had not shown up the week beginning 16 March. Parents were already ahead of the politicians.

It turned out that the coronavirus was ahead of us too, personally as well as professionally and strategically. Neil, one of those on the phone, had developed a fever and dry cough and was isolating at home. Several other advisers ended up falling sick around the same time – they had all been sitting at one end of the table in the Victoria Street basement meeting room at a previous SAGE meeting.

After the 18 March meeting, Demis emailed me saying he had heard that the virus had reached Victoria Street. Did I have any symptoms, he asked, and should he start worrying?

❋ ❋ ❋

That afternoon, the Prime Minister addressed the nation. He announced that schools would close at the end of the week until further notice, except for vulnerable children and the children of key workers.

The day after, on 19 March, the health secretary Matt Hancock introduced the Coronavirus Bill to the UK Parliament. The legislation would give police sweeping powers to detain and isolate members of the public, to close ports and airports and, if necessary, stop people meeting and gathering. It loosened restrictions on retired doctors so they could come back to work without jeopardising pension rights. A COBR meeting was scheduled for Friday 20 March 2020. Astonishingly, the PM reportedly skipped it.

It was not until the next SAGE meeting, on Monday 23 March, after ten wasted days, that reality would hit those in power: the epidemic was on a runaway trajectory.

At that meeting, the modellers offered a chilling, two-page consensus statement on how the rapidly expanding outbreak would evolve. The number of confirmed coronavirus patients entering intensive care was doubling every three to five days, meaning that hospitals in the capital would be overrun by end of March. The statement ran: 'It is very likely that we will see ICU capacity in London breached by the end of the month, even if additional measures are put in place today.' Breaches outside London would come one or two weeks later. None of this was a surprise to those who had been paying attention in the three previous SAGE meetings.

The virus was also probably more transmissible than originally suspected, a critical fact that had lain obscured in the early, fuzzy epidemiological data. The statement continued: 'The observed rapid increase in ICU admissions is consistent with a higher reproduction number than 2.4 ... [We] cannot rule out it being higher than 3.' That meant that every infected person was potentially passing it to three or more people. Seasonal flu has a reproduction number of about 1.4.

The take-home message, yet again, was that the UK was in a dire place. We did not know how many cases were accruing in the community, because testing could not be ramped up enough to keep pace and was therefore confined to hospitals; it was too early to gauge how well people were cutting social contacts after the government announcement on 18 March; those unknowns made it hard to figure out computationally what might happen when school closures were thrown into the mix.

Shopping data, though, offered a pointer to the mood of the country. Consumer spending on food and medicines was rocketing: people were stockpiling and supermarkets were rationing toilet roll and pasta to stop shelves being stripped bare.

❋ ❋ ❋

Those deafening messages from the SAGE meetings of 13, 16, 18 and 23 March – that the country was racing dangerously up the epidemic curve, and that those in power needed to put the brakes on – finally struck home at the heart of government. At 8.30pm that night, Boris Johnson addressed the nation to announce that a legal stay-at-home order would be put in place immediately. SAGE did not advise closing borders to all countries; given that the UK epidemic was mostly seeded by travellers from Europe, the UK would have had to totally close its borders (including to Europe) by 1 February at the latest, to have altered the course of the epidemic. Even with hindsight, I do not think that would have been feasible.

The new restrictions meant people would be unable to leave home except for one of four reasons: to travel to and from work if work could not be done from home; to exercise once a day; to buy food and medicines; and to seek medical care. Shops selling non-essential goods would shut and gatherings of more than two people who did not live together would be banned. People were warned to keep two metres away from people they did not live with. Weddings, parties, religious services would stop, but funerals could still go ahead. SAGE, like so many other working groups around the world, switched to using Zoom.

The most at-risk groups, including those with health conditions and the over-70s, needed to stay indoors for 12 weeks. This new way of life would be strictly policed. The Coronavirus Act 2020 came into law by the end of that week.

The UK was finally going into the kind of lockdown that Italy, France, Spain and Belgium had already enacted.* As I noted in my 24 March update to Wellcome colleagues:

The UK COVID19 policy finally aligned with global efforts – I do not believe you will hear the term 'Natural herd immunity is our strategy' again from UKG.

But it had taken ten days to act – during which the doubling time of the epidemic was perhaps five days or less. The decision not to act sooner was wrong and undoubtedly cost lives. In June 2020, Neil Ferguson told the House of Commons Science and Technology Select Committee that locking down one week earlier would have halved the death toll. By the time Neil spoke, around 40,000 people in the UK had lost their lives to coronavirus. That was, on the face of it, an appalling miscalculation: 20,000 lives swapped for an extra week of liberty. Postponing intervention against contagion is a false economy and a drain on freedom: a country that shuts down later stays closed for longer – and risks losing the trust of its citizens that the State can protect them.

As the UK was entering its lockdown, China was seeing the fruits of its own policies. Up until 24 March 2020, the city of Wuhan had not seen a new coronavirus case for five days. There was other good news: the Moderna Covid-19 vaccine trial was up and running, and several clinical trials to test out potential treatments were underway across 40 countries. But, I noted to Wellcome colleagues in one of my confidential updates, the global numbers were rocketing:

65 Days for 1–100,000 confirmed cases

11 Days for 100,001–200,000 confirmed cases

---

* Italy went into a national lockdown on 9 March; Spain on 16 March; France on 17 March; and Belgium on 18 March.

4 Days for 200,001–300,000 confirmed cases

2 Days to reach 400,000 confirmed cases

Now confirmed in every country

As March neared its end, the virus reached the corridors of power. On 27 March 2020, at the end of the first week of lockdown, both the health secretary Matt Hancock and prime minister Boris Johnson revealed they had tested positive for coronavirus. Hancock suffered relatively mild synptoms but Johnson was not so fortunate. On 6 April, the PM was rushed to intensive care and was given oxygen during the journey to St Thomas's Hospital, which lies across Westminster Bridge from the Houses of Parliament. The foreign secretary, Dominic Raab, was assigned to deputise for him.

※ ※ ※

The immediate threat in March going into April was that hospitals would be overwhelmed, that what happened in Italy would happen to us. The UK had to scale up capacity, as China had done so impressively. In the space of nine days, east London's Excel Centre, one of the country's biggest conference venues, was converted into a temporary field hospital. Two other so-called Nightingale hospitals were opened later in Manchester and Birmingham. They were impressive up to a point: they lacked the trained staff to operate properly.

But, even as new trenches were dug, we were still fighting an unseen enemy. Testing was being dangerously outpaced by transmission and was proving to be the Achilles heel of the UK response. Public Health England was doing around 10,000 per week by 11 March. By comparison, Germany was doing 500,000 a week, some in drive-through centres. Countries further afield, such as Singapore and South Korea, were also mounting impressive epidemic containment operations.

In April, it became obvious the virus was spreading in hospitals. But we were hamstrung; without firing up testing capacity it was impossible to gauge what was going on in hospitals and care homes. And the levers were still not budging. No matter how much SAGE advised that such testing was central to any strategy, advisers had no operational power or oversight to make it happen.

With high rates of nosocomial (hospital/care home) transmission, the obvious thing to do would have been to test all staff, including cleaners and ambulance drivers, so they could isolate if infected. But testing also presented a Faustian bargain: do we test everyone working in hospitals, plus patients and staff, knowing that maybe 25 per cent of the workforce would have to isolate and the NHS would collapse? Or do we essentially turn a blind eye?

That blindness lit the touchpaper for the devastating epidemic in hospitals and care homes. Patients with the virus were discharged, untested, from hospital back into sometimes barely regulated institutional settings, where poorly paid carers work across multiple care homes. Often, hospitals had little choice but to send patients back to care homes; they had been instructed to clear beds for the coming storm.

The minutes of the SAGE meeting of 5 May 2020 painted a disturbing picture of 'three separate but interacting epidemics: in the community; in hospitals; and in care homes'. Hospitals and care homes became the biggest block to loosening restrictions, even though six weeks of lockdown had pushed the reproduction number down, as hoped. R was now lying between 0.5 and 0.9; the outbreak was, the figures suggested, shrinking.

But lockdowns alone cannot get a society back to normality: as I never tire of saying, they do not change the fundamentals of a virus or a pandemic. Staying indoors does not alter a pathogen's transmissibility or ability to wreak harm; it just takes susceptible people out of circulation. When a lockdown ends, those people go back into circulation again. Without a vaccine or other measures in place, untying restrictions increases social contacts and transmissions rise. If restrictions eased and R shot up to 3 again, we would find ourselves back at square one, with an epidemic racing exponentially out of control as it did in late March 2020. Science – vaccines, drugs, testing – was the only exit strategy.

As SAGE noted that day and previously, the UK needed a test, trace and isolate system (TTI). It had to be in place before restrictions were lifted, because TTI works best when infections are low to begin with. It is a bit like rigging up a system to detect forest fires: a small flare-up is easily spied against a quiet background but not amid a raging blaze. TTI is a textbook recommendation in public health and countries like Germany and South Korea were running it smoothly. Why couldn't the UK?

Ministers decided it should be run centrally and, on 7 May, Baroness Dido Harding was appointed as its unpaid chair. It was a grave error. Health secretary Matt Hancock praised her 'significant experience in healthcare and fantastic leadership', but I could not see what skills she brought to the role. She chaired the regulator NHS Improvement but she had no extensive experience of public health.

Some of her comments to select committees since then have done nothing to soften my opinion. She claimed that nobody could have predicted the surge in September 2020, at the beginning of the second wave. That surge was obvious and had even been modelled: cases were creeping upwards just before schools opened. As Timothy Gowers says, epidemiology is sometimes about grasping basic maths.

SAGE concluded later in the year that Test and Trace, launched in late May, delivered only a marginal benefit, even though many talented people dedicated great effort to trying to tackle its shortcomings. Despite the PM claiming it would be world-beating, it was not really functional nor anywhere near the capacity needed to make a difference. Contact tracing needs to reach 80 per cent of an infected person's contacts within 48 hours to make inroads into an epidemic. The reality was closer to 50 per cent.

Centralising the TTI, and bypassing local authorities, was a mistake. As anyone who has ever worked in diseases knows: all epidemics are local. Local authorities around the UK housed regional public health teams who knew their communities well and were used to contact tracing for outbreaks of food poisoning and sexually transmitted diseases.

A related problem around that time was the NHSX app, integral to the TTI effort. Apple and Google had offered to help to deliver a tracing app, but the government insisted on keeping everything in-house. I had spoken to people like Regina Dugan, who runs Wellcome Leap, our futuristic research arm, about this approach.* Regina has previously worked at Facebook and Google, and the view of people with her expertise was that any attempt to go it alone was likely to fail. That proved to be true, but the go-it-alone mentality persisted for far too long, to nobody's benefit.

---

* Wellcome Leap is meant to be a global ARPA for health. ARPA was the Advanced Research Projects Agency set up by the US in 1958, in worried response to the surprise launch of Sputnik by the Soviet Union the year before.

A similar lack of focus plagued thinking on ventilators: worries in March 2020 that 8,000 NHS ventilators might be insufficient led to a call for British manufacturers to design and build new basic ones at speed. Companies with no history of making medical devices, like Rolls-Royce and Dyson, were recruited to the cause. The specs changed in April, as did treatment plans, and companies that were already making such machines to regulatory standards complained they had been sidelined. Many projects were quietly dropped and the government's order for Dyson ventilators was cancelled.

There were random decisions, about this app or that product, plucked from the sky that did not seem informed by any knowledge of public health. These ideas would be flavour of the month until they crashed and burned. It was the kind of haphazard, hour-by-hour decision-making in a crisis that wastes time, money, resources and emotional energy. Despite the best efforts of many fantastic civil servants, there was too little standing back and strategising.

The atmosphere of chaos made the government vulnerable to what looked like racketeering. I remember sitting in a Downing Street meeting hosted by Boris Johnson and being surrounded by some very good diagnostics companies who were trying to do the right thing, but also snake oil salesmen pushing rapid tests which were just useless. Everybody was just scrambling to buy whatever testing they could. There were arbitrary decisions to spend large amounts of money to order things even though everyone, including PHE, knew they were rubbish. It sometimes felt as if I had strayed on a set for *The Third Man*, that fantastic Carol Reed film of a Graham Greene novel, which features a black market for penicillin. At one point during April, I contacted Number 10 asking them to stop the government ordering rapid tests that were both useless and a massive distraction. At that time, there were no good rapid tests.

What was missing in March, April and May was calm strategic thinking. One bright spot was the appointment in April of Paul Deighton, the chief executive behind London's 2012 Olympics, to solve the PPE shortage. He came in and sorted it all out very quietly behind the scenes. Another was Kate Bingham, chair of the Vaccine Taskforce, whose brio and competence stood out against a background of systemic mediocrity. It was all too common a pattern: individuals were incredibly able and willing, but were frustrated by the chaos, bureaucracy and lack of strategic direction.

I sent a message into Number 10 that there should be a bunch of people unshackled from day-to-day responsibility and ruthlessly focused on the next phase of the pandemic response:

This needs a dedicated team sent away to design what is needed … testing, isolation, contact tracing, logistics, data etc – a military style campaign that may last June–September. Get that wrong like PPE, testing fiasco, and it will be a disaster…

❋ ❋ ❋

That drawn-out, stressful period also saw two SAGE attendees embroiled in more personal dramas. On 27 March 2020, against lockdown rules, Dominic Cummings, chief adviser to prime minister Boris Johnson, drove himself and his family to his in-laws in Durham while possibly infected. He has since told a parliamentary committee that he did this because he and his family received death threats – but, whatever the circumstances, it was a disastrous mistake for someone in a public position.

Cummings refused to resign – and Johnson, who himself left hospital on 12 April after recovering from Covid, did not sack him. Cummings gave a press conference defending himself in the Rose Garden at the PM's residence. Whatever his story, he knew the rules and his actions sent a powerful signal that we were not all in this together, that the laws were different depending on who you were. As Jonathan Van-Tam, England's deputy chief medical officer, said at the time, the rules applied to everyone. Public adherence depended on this basic principle, as the behavioural experts made clear.

The second transgression hit closer to home and made me realise how much scientists had become figures of hate. On 5 May 2020, it was revealed that Neil had broken lockdown rules. A married woman with whom he was having a relationship was seen visiting his flat. Details of his private life were splashed all over the *Daily Telegraph*, and he only learned of it on the day of publication. He resigned from SAGE immediately (he still contributes to SPI-M and NERVTAG). Neil explained that, having recovered from Covid-19, he thought he was immune.

Neil would be the first to accept that he made a mistake and I know he regrets what happened. But the vitriol in the newspapers directed at him, and some of the comments about him from ministers, seemed deliberately designed to undermine both him as an individual and his science, and SAGE by implication. The libertarians hated him because they saw his numbers, wrongly, as the driving force behind lockdowns, even though he was just one among several modellers.

So they borrowed from the playbook used by the tobacco lobby and climate change sceptics: first, undermine the individual, then undermine the data and the advice. Dig out other scientists ready to give a so-called expert view that is diametrically opposed. The aim is to cast enough doubt on the science to sow public confusion. Presenting data and graphs of likely scenarios with confidence intervals was the right thing to do but it enabled critics to seize on the extremes, especially projections, to discredit perfectly reasonable central estimates.

Neil regrets what he calls the 'hyper-polarisation' of the media, which saw him become a bête noire of newspapers such as the *Wall Street Journal*, *Telegraph* and the *Mail*: 'The trend of choosing what to believe and what not to believe has been amplified in the pandemic. We've always had our fair share of conspiracy theorists and others on the fringes of the internet but what has been particularly disappointing is that media outlets have taken an avowedly political perspective. Their editorial departments seem to be less interested in the truth than in a political agenda and cherrypick things accordingly. It's been shocking to see that in the UK.'

Neil admits the episode 'took an emotional toll. I didn't do much work for a week and, when I came back, I stopped working 18-hour days and began to take some weekends off. I think it's had an emotional toll on everyone. It's just exhausting working flat out for long periods of time.'

Patrick Vallance has been kind and supportive, Neil says, and he has also attended some voluntary group sessions set up to support SAGE members. He dislikes being a public figure and winces at his nickname of 'Professor Lockdown'. Neil adds: 'I've only been recognised in the street a couple of times, both times by people who were nice.'

SAGE advisers, all unpaid but serving gladly out of a sense of civic duty, were receiving a lot of media attention and, as Neil's experience showed, much of it was hostile, even though we were slogging through nights and weekends to make sure the advice was ready to feed into government. We were designated key workers. We were also trying to do our day jobs.

We were offered pastoral care, advice on personal security and given a hotline to call to report any concerns. I used it when my children were trolled on social media. Just because they share my surname does not make them fair game. The personal abuse is relentless.

John was also disturbed by the fact Neil had essentially been spied on. He had his own run-in with the *Telegraph*, with a reporter who seemed to be fishing for stories about conflicts of interest. John holds an EU grant to work with Johnson & Johnson on an Ebola vaccine, and his partner works for a pharmaceutical company. John remembers: 'The reporter was asking me how many shares my partner owned and insinuating I was taking money from Johnson & Johnson. I had already declared everything and eventually they gave up.' On the day the story about Neil was published, John stopped cycling to his university office and switched to working from home.

On 10 May 2020, I updated my colleagues with my worries about the apparent lifting of lockdown. That day, the PM had urged people who could not work from home to return to the office while avoiding public transport. Lifting lockdown was a prospect that alarmed SAGE, given how high infections were still running:

Europe and North America are now running a fairly ad hoc experiment on the lifting of restrictions. UK will be one of the last countries able to put this in place … the consequence of poor decisions made end of January and during February

Until the epidemics in care homes, prisons and hospitals are brought under control infection rates in UK will remain stubbornly high and the ability to lift restrictions further will be limited

This has been the advice of SAGE for at least 2 months…

The rest of May felt like a struggle to keep the floodgates shut. R was hovering stubbornly around 0.7–1.0. It needed to stay below 1 for the epidemic to shrink. But TTI was not properly in place and the UK was racking up as many as 9,000 new cases every day. Loosening restrictions while infections were running that high would quickly swamp the system.

Schools would have a phased reopening from 1 June 2020, with non-essential retail following on 15 June. SAGE feared that multiple sectors – schools, retail, hospitality – would all be flung open in quick succession or all at once, rather than spacing them out to test the effect of each restriction on transmission. That would throw multiple canisters of fuel on to a viral fire that was waiting to be stoked again.

In pressing to reopen, the PM might have been trying to meet his own timetable. Back on 19 March, Johnson declared that the UK could 'turn the tide on coronavirus' in 12 weeks. The deadline of 11 June was looming. SAGE believed that data, not dates, should set the timetable. Despite claims by the government that it was 'following the science', it was not. As in March, it was treading its own less cautious route under the cover of science.

On 31 May, a day that saw more than 1,000 coronavirus infections added to the national tally, I spelled out to my Wellcome colleagues what a mess the UK was in:

People may have lost their trust in authority.

No other country in Europe has lifted their restrictions with the case numbers UK has now. All countries had total daily new cases in the 100s when they lifted restrictions and all had more robust surveillance in place.

It is absolutely right that the decision to lift restrictions is a political decision.

What is not right is that politicians claim that the decision has been made on the basis of SAGE scientific advice.

What infuriated me was the lack of honesty with the public. SAGE advice was unanimous: infections were high, TTI was crawling along at a snail's pace, the app was a disaster, and any release, let alone multiple loosenings, would trigger a rise in cases that would be tough to track and contain.

Ministers were not following the science, even if they said they were. Governments owe it to people to be clear about when they are following advice and when they are rejecting it. They must shoulder responsibility for the decisions and be upfront about the possible trade-offs. The public should have been warned that cases would rise as restrictions eased. Instead, they were led to believe the epidemic was over.

Perhaps ministers were hoping that science would ride to the rescue. Clinical trials of several Covid-19 vaccines, including a home-grown one by Oxford University and AstraZeneca, were underway; there were even rumours that the Oxford vaccine might be ready by September. On 16 June, there was a terrific therapeutic breakthrough courtesy of the RECOVERY trial coordinated by Oxford University and using the amazing clinical network in the NHS built up over many years. It reported that a cheap steroid called dexamethasone could cut the chances of death among the sickest Covid-19 patients by a third.

※ ※ ※

These were high points amid the gathering gloom, particularly the RECOVERY trial because I remember the wonderful moment it was born: on the number 18 bus.

I had caught the train from Oxford to London and then jumped on the 18 bus from Marylebone station to escape the rain. Martin Landray happened to be on the same train, happened to get on the same bus and happened to be heading the same way: to the Wellcome Trust.

Martin is an epidemiologist and professor of medicine at Oxford University who spends a lot of time thinking about how to measure the benefits (or otherwise) of drugs and treatments. Six months earlier, Martin had started advising Wellcome on how to make clinical trials all over the world easier and quicker to carry out. Trials are notoriously complicated, slow and bureaucratic to set up: the guidelines drawn up by the International Council for Harmonisation of Technical Requirements for Pharmaceuticals for Human Use run to more than 60 pages. In many ways, with the paperwork and protocols, clinical trials can end up hobbling research rather than adding to it.

It was surreal: I remember standing downstairs with Martin on this crowded bus talking as quietly as we could about the wave of disease that was about to hit the UK. We were whispering to avoid alarming passengers, and eventually got off the bus early so we could have a proper conversation. Humanity had nothing in the medicine cabinet. And yet patients were already coming into hospitals, some of whom would fall seriously ill and die. I asked him how quickly clinical trials could be set up to test potential therapies for Covid-19 and said that Wellcome would help to fund it.

But I also knew, after Ebola, that the usual grind of a trial would not work in the middle of a chaotic epidemic. That was why ISARIC (International Severe and Acute Respiratory and Emerging Infection Consortium) had been set up years earlier, along with the WHO Blueprint and CEPI. The consortium had a stripped-down how-to guide showing how to get clinical trials up and running quickly and had already proved its worth during the Ebola epidemic. Peter Horby, now the director of ISARIC and a former colleague of mine in Vietnam, was at Oxford University and had already started trials in China with Bin Cao. During January and February, Peter had also started planning UK trials and shortlisting potential therapies. I put Martin in touch with him.

The rest is medical history. Days later, Martin and Peter finished hammering out the terms of the RECOVERY trial (Randomised Evaluation of Covid-19 Therapies), allowing hospitals all over the UK to simply go to a website, enrol a patient, input some minimal data and then be told which drug to give. Within nine days of the bus journey, the first patient was signed up.

Given that some of the worst symptoms of the disease seemed to be associated with an out-of-control immune reaction, the first drugs they chose to test were therapies known to calm the immune system down, a potentially risky approach when patients are fighting for their lives. But the sheer scale of the trial, potentially open to anyone admitted to an NHS hospital with Covid-19, meant doctors and patients could have confidence in the results. Within about three months, humanity finally had something – dexamethasone – in the medicine cabinet. It was not a cure-all but it could save some lives. It has already saved a million lives and will save millions more. As importantly, it has shown what does not work, including hydroxychloroquine (touted early on as a cure).

�֍ ✷ ✷

Still, we were a long way from safety. I longed to be wrong but I could almost see the rebound coming over the horizon. Cases were no longer falling but plateauing.

My best estimate, I added in the 31 May update, was that cases would begin climbing in England in late June or early July. Infections indeed reached their lowest, the Office for National Statistics estimated, between 22 and 26 June, and hospital cases were at their lowest in early July, reflecting the time lag between infection and serious symptoms. This is not brilliant forecasting on my part but plain and simple epidemiology.

I wrote to my Wellcome colleagues, somewhat fearfully, that I was 'concerned that everyone has interpreted 'lockdown is over''. That was certainly the mood music. Pubs and restaurants threw open their doors on 4 July; newspapers celebrated the UK's 'Independence Day' from the virus. On 3 August, the 'Eat Out To Help Out' scheme began. Diners would receive hefty discounts on meals served in venues but not for takeaways. John renamed it 'Eat Out to Help the Virus Out'. Mike Ferguson at Wellcome called it 'Eat Out to Spread It About'. By then, the UK Covid-19 death toll exceeded 46,000.

Against a background of high prevalence, doubts over TTI and with an R only just below 1, the collective signalling was unmistakable: Independence Day, eat out to help out, get back to work, we're behind the worst of it, the sun is shining, live without fear.

The effect was to create a tinderbox. Case numbers started rising through the months of July and August 2020. Minutes of a SAGE meeting held on 6 August noted: 'Considering all available data, it is likely that incidence is static or may be increasing, meaning R may be above 1 in England.'

Later that month, infections began rising dramatically in Birmingham, particularly in the South Asian community. Throughout August, there were concerns that not enough infected people were self-isolating, because they feared losing pay, and that TTI was not fast or comprehensive enough to stem spread.

The reopening of schools in September piled on more tinder. The rise in infections would be carried into winter, as people came into closer proximity. Europe looked to be a harbinger of what was to come: in France, in the last week of August, numbers of infections rose daily: first 5,000 a day, then 6,000, then 7,000, followed by an influx of patients to intensive care units in Paris. I was having conversations with specialists across the Channel, knowing that wherever France went, the UK would follow. Hospitalisations and deaths would come to the UK once more, too.

As case numbers rose, wishful thinking and optimism bias returned. It is tempting to see a small flick upwards in the numbers and think, 'maybe it's just a blip and it will go down again'. So begins a futile hope, without any evidence, that perhaps natural immunity has developed and things will be different this time. You desperately hope what you have just been through will never come back.

Sometimes, hope is not enough.

7

*Are we complicit in the outcomes?**

31 AUGUST 2020

Known global cases: 24,854,140
Global deaths: 838,924
UK cases: 332,756; UK deaths: 41,498
(within 28 days of a positive Covid-19 test)

ON 31 AUGUST 2020, exactly eight months after the first cases were reported to the WHO, I guided my inner circle at Wellcome around the globe in one of my confidential updates. My personal estimate of the true number of global cases was between 200 and 300 million.

The epicentre for the accelerating pandemic is now South Asia – India, Bangladesh, Nepal, Pakistan.

USA/Canada: The epidemic has shifted from major population centres (New York, Florida, Texas, California) to less densely populated mid-West America and Canada ...

---

* 'The central moral dilemma: does staying in an advisory role mean being complicit in the outcomes of bad decisions?' (author – p.176).

Central and South America: Brazil (Rio/SP), Mexico (City) are at or just beyond their peak incidence but as in USA this epidemic is now spreading to more rural areas...

Africa: I believe is still at the start of transmission, protected a little by demographics, climate and lower connectivity, but remains very vulnerable...

China, Japan, Korea and South East Asia

Most cases in China are now in people travelling into China from other countries and there remain very strict control measures in place...

Vietnam remains under very draconian local or national controls.

Singapore has essentially controlled the epidemic except within their migrant worker community...

Australia increased cases in Victoria, but so far not nationally. NZ still very much under control with isolation. Pacific Islands seeing increased cases.

Europe

We are clearly entering a new phase as we transition from summer into autumn…

The spread into rural areas around the world was inevitable but concerning: people in the countryside tend to be older than city dwellers and healthcare is patchier. It also meant the virus was widening its geographical footprint.

Just two weeks after that update, cases in India rocketed up to 100,000 a day, reflecting an easing of very tight lockdown restrictions that came into effect in March. The Indian Council of Medical Research had promised a Covid-19 vaccine would be ready by 15 August 2020, India's Independence Day. The date came and went, another example of optimism bias by a populist leader, this time Indian prime minister Narendra Modi (though it would be unfair to tar Modi with the same anti-science brush as other populist leaders, such as Trump and Jair Bolsonaro in Brazil).

Even if India had missed its own self-imposed deadline, Russia and China were racing ahead with their own government-backed vaccine development programmes. In August 2020, Russia approved its home-grown Covid-19 vaccine, Sputnik–V, but released very little data publicly, raising scepticism about its efficacy and safety. The final phase of clinical trials, Phase 3, which constitute the large-scale test of how a vaccine works in the real world, had not yet concluded.

Medical regulators that green-light vaccines for public use are meant to be free of political interference; while I was confident of this with the UK, Europe and China, I was less sure about Russia. With a vaccine named in homage to a Soviet-era space race, the expedited approval seemed more of a political triumph than a scientific one.

A cloud, meanwhile, was gathering over the Oxford/AstraZeneca vaccine, which used a different adenovirus in its formulation. In early September, trials of AZ1222 were paused in multiple countries after a volunteer fell ill with symptoms of transverse myelitis, a (usually) temporary neurological condition. Such pauses are common: it takes time to assess whether volunteers who fall sick during clinical trials have suffered a coincidental but unrelated bout of ill health or a genuine adverse effect as a result of the trial.

It was critical to maintain public trust in the vaccines; getting out of the pandemic depended on people's willingness to take them. At the time, I guessed the jabs would be around 40–60 per cent effective, hovering around the threshold of 50 per cent required by the WHO for approval. I would have

been staggered had I been told that some (pre-variant) effica-
cies would exceed 90 per cent. I am still staggered now.

✴ ✴ ✴

Back in April 2020, as the pandemic was gathering pace
around the world, Richard Hatchett from CEPI kindly roped
me into emails and telephone calls drawing up a grand plan
to accelerate discussions on vaccine development. The emails
were coordinated by Richard Danzig, an inspiring figure: a
former secretary of the US Navy under Bill Clinton, adviser
to Barack Obama and, as the other Richard called him, a
'biodefence intellectual'. These were energising conversations, spurring us to think ambitiously about what could be
achieved: a Manhattan Project for vaccines and drugs.

Instead of the usual 12- to 18-month schedule, which was
itself seen as wishful thinking, Danzig felt the vaccine time-
line could be crushed to six months. The plan was to reach
out to major governments around the world, such as the US,
India, China and Japan. Danzig could already see in March
2020 that the obstacles blocking an exit from the pandemic
would not be the science but the physical supply of vaccines,
from the manufacturing lines down to the availability of
glass vials.

Danzig understood that, if the world wanted vaccines by
the end of 2020, it would have to start getting the financing
and other pieces of the puzzle, such as manufacturing,
scaled up quickly – and all over the world. The calls were
an attempt to galvanise the whole community to throw
everything at this, to point out that the costs of doing it were
trivial compared to the costs of not doing it. Too often, the
first thing we ask about a problem is how much it will cost to
fix. This was the opposite: what did the world need to do to

get out of the pandemic? It was diagnostics, treatments and vaccines. The cost was secondary.

Danzig's idea of an international Manhattan Project did not get off the ground, but elements were absorbed into Operation Warp Speed, the $18-billion US project to deliver 300 million doses of vaccines by January 2021. Another spin-off was an EU-pledging conference on 4 May 2020. The goal for this was to get pledges of $8 billion. Looking back, it was too low but that is the dance of global health: you don't want to ask for a stupid figure that nobody will support, but it means you will always get less than you need. In retrospect, I wish we had just said, 'Look the pandemic is going to be awful, it's going to keep going round and round and if you invest $100 billion now, in a year's time you'll be glad you did.' Instead, in April and May 2020, many countries thought the pandemic was behind them. In that context, a request for $100 billion to manufacture vaccines that did not yet exist would fall on deaf ears. Still, in June 2021 the WHO and World Bank pleaded for $50 billion as the world continued to suffer. Imagine where we would have been if we had had that money in May 2020.

Even if the US, Russia and China were on track to sort out vaccines for their own citizens, there was no guarantee there would be enough doses to span the globe. Vaccines needed to be available everywhere, not just to countries able to develop and manufacture them or rich ones able to buy them in. Billions of doses would be required, including in remote areas and in conflict zones. Nobody could be safe until everyone was safe.

※ ※ ※

By then, the WHO had already set up something called the ACT-Accelerator. 'ACT' stands for 'Access to Covid-19

Tools', and by 'tools', we meant all the things that help to stop diseases in their tracks: tests, treatments, PPE, oxygen and vaccines. The sole purpose of the accelerator was to bring an end to the pandemic as quickly as possible by speeding up the development of all these necessities, then making them and despatching them to as many countries in the world as possible. All these tools would be needed everywhere in order to halt spread.

As summer wore on and rumours swirled that potentially effective vaccines would come on stream in the autumn or winter, the chink in the master plan to vaccinate the world became disturbingly plain: not every country had a supply line.

Both China and Russia planned to use their own vaccines to protect their own citizens; both also pledged doses to a total of around 30 nations (both offered plentiful doses to countries in Africa, in what has been interpreted as 'vaccine diplomacy'). Another 60 countries were eligible for help with vaccines through GAVI, which in usual times brings lifesaving vaccines to some of the poorest nations, particularly to children.

That still left around 130 countries, including the UK, Singapore, Japan and Norway, with no obvious access to doses. Several of them, including the UK and Japan, set up their own vaccine task forces, to negotiate with manufacturers to procure supplies for their own citizens. While I was initially disappointed that the UK had opted out of the European Union procurement scheme, the UK's Vaccine Taskforce*, led by Kate Bingham, has been one of the standout successes of the country's pandemic response. While I don't like saying it, it was the best possible example

---

* Declaration of interest: I am a member of the Vaccine Taskforce.

of British exceptionalism: approaching a challenge with a mix of urgency, risk-taking and pragmatism. I am sure many in Europe wish the same approach had been brought to bear on behalf of the bloc.

Not every country, though, has the expertise or funds to assemble its own vaccines portfolio. In July 2020, Singapore convened a meeting of around 160 countries that led to COVAX (one overlooked pandemic risk is the spread of baffling acronyms). COVAX, which stands for the 'Covid-19 Vaccines Global Access Facility', is an all-out effort to make sure all countries can get hold of vaccines regardless of their ability to pay.

It operates like a buyers club and insurance market: countries throw money into a pool and COVAX cuts deals with vaccine manufacturers on the buyers' behalf. The payments give COVAX bargaining power, but also enable investment into a range of vaccine projects to smooth their delivery.

Countries signing up to COVAX were still able to strike up their own bilateral deals with manufacturers – as the UK did. COVAX, by backing a wide range of vaccine projects, offered a safety net if none of the vaccine bets in national portfolios came through. COVAX has had considerable international buy-in: China, India and the US have come on board. The majority of the world's countries are participants, either as donors or participants or both.

Humanitarian agencies such as the International Red Cross and Red Crescent will be able to apply for doses too; these doses are destined for refugees and those living in hard-to-reach areas such as conflict zones. Ultimately, the plan was for COVAX to secure two billion doses by the end of 2021. It has so far raised $6 billion but needs another $2 billion to meet its target for 2021.

Even so, there is a fundamental difficulty: rich countries, even those which have paid into COVAX, now monopolise vaccine supply. The UK ordered five times as many doses as it needs, while on 1 June 2021 the WHO reported that low-income countries had received less than 1 per cent of vaccines administered. Over-ordering is the right approach in a high risk situation, because none are guaranteed to work. However, countries now need to share some of those doses with countries that desperately need them.

I hope COVAX is able to fulfil what it was set up to do: to bring vaccines to everyone, irrespective of ability to pay. COVAX became one of four pillars, or components, of the ACT-Accelerator, specifically covering vaccines. The other three pillars cover diagnostics and testing, treatments, and the strengthening of health systems.

The ACT-Accelerator (or, more fully, the 'Access to Covid-19 Tools Accelerator') is a valuable organisation that has been set up from scratch at breakneck speed. There has been a dizzying pulling together of activities, from basic science and new vaccines, to funding via the World Bank, and then delivery and implementation which is the hardest bit, of course. It negotiates contracts with manufacturers; organises distribution and sorts out the logistics, including cold chains.

I was involved with setting up the accelerator. And, to begin with, it was a nightmare.

❋ ❋ ❋

How do you tackle the worst pandemic you have ever seen at the fastest possible pace? That was the idea behind the ACT-Accelerator. It meant persuading some of the biggest names in global health to work together for one purpose: to end the acute phase of the pandemic (which means bringing transmission under control) as quickly as humanly possible.

Even though Geneva was the right place to host such an important international effort, I was initially sceptical that it should be driven by the WHO. Trump had threatened to withdraw from the agency and was kicking it at every opportunity, and China had effectively ended up defending it. I feared the accelerator, central to the global effort to end the pandemic, and for which Wellcome bore some responsibility for the therapeutics part, would become a political football.

I argued about it over the phone with Tedros, the WHO director general, and his chief of staff, Bernhard Schwartlander. I thought it needed a completely independent secretariat, to avoid being closely allied to any of the partners: the WHO, World Bank, Unitaid, Global Fund, FIND, GAVI (also known as the Vaccine Alliance), CEPI, Wellcome Trust, and the Gates Foundation. It was a robust conversation and by the end of it Tedros had persuaded me that a WHO hub seemed the least worst option. I lost the argument, but he was right and I was wrong. It was launched within weeks, in April 2020, and has been been reasonably successful.

Tedros remained true to his word about the WHO being the convenor but never the controller: he attends all the ACT-Accelerator meetings, but has never chaired one. Bruce Aylward, a colleague of Tedros who brings it all together, has put incredible energy – and the hours to match – into making the ACT-Accelerator work in exactly the rigorous, independent manner I was fighting for.

After launching it, we then had to thrash out which non-WHO figures could lead it. That too happened in a whirlwind of teleconference calls and phone calls. The first six months, from about July to December 2020, were jointly masterminded by GAVI's board chair Dr Ngozi Okonjo-Iweala, an economist and former finance minister of Nigeria who later became the first woman and first African to become director general of the World Trade Organization; and Andrew Witty, the former chief executive of GlaxoSmithKline. They made a real power couple: Ngozi with her financial background, and Andrew a trusted voice in the pharmaceutical industry who knew about R&D manufacturing. Both made it clear they would only do the job until December 2020.

Leading something like this is unbelievably intense. The accelerator brought within its orbit a coalition of organisations that were unused to sharing the spotlight, with big egos jostling for space. I don't necessarily mean personal egos but organisational egos attached to big names and big brands.

The NGO sector does not work together as well as it could, partly because of the way it is funded. Every few years, organisations have to go cap in hand to governments for money. To do that, they have to be front and centre of everything, hogging the show. Sharing the limelight does not come naturally.

That is why the chairs played such a critical role: keeping a coalition like that together means bridging divides, soothing egos, jollying people along and putting an arm round people when they are feeling down. Ngozi and Andrew were brilliant, but happened to step down just as the pressure was building.

Everyone could see where that pressure was coming from. By September 2020, it was becoming clear that vaccines were going to be in short supply, as were treatments and diagnostic tests. There were going to be shortfalls of oxygen and PPE, too. I became the interim chair in December 2020, but was not the right person for the job. It needed someone with political savvy. I was terrified that the ACT-Accelerator was going to fall apart. I pestered Tedros and Bruce constantly, texting them almost every day, to get Ngozi and Andrew's successors in place.

And then, almost out of nowhere, Tedros floated the idea of approaching Carl Bildt, the former prime minister of Sweden and a peacemaker in the Balkans. Tedros was foreign minister in Ethiopia and is plugged into that broader international political scene. He had Carl's number.

It was an inspired suggestion: in 2021, ending the pandemic is no longer a scientific problem but a political one. It needs a statesman like Carl, with his track record of brokering complex political deals, to do what only a handful of people around the world can do: just pick up the phone to anybody at any time, knowing someone will answer. I handed over the ACT-Accelerator to him at the end of March 2021, and he will soon be joined by a chair from the Global South.

The last year has been an eye-opener for me. I thought, probably like most people, that the world works through official or formal channels but much of it operates through private phone calls and messaging apps. Whether it is teen-agers in Oxford chatting to each other, or the DG of the World Health Organization reaching out to a former prime minister of Sweden, the conversation probably starts with a pinged message.

❋ ❋ ❋

While things were moving frantically on the international front in the summer of 2020, with hopes building for several successful vaccines, the situation in the UK was deteriorating swiftly. The autumn of 2020 was, without doubt, the lowest point for me during the pandemic. I seriously considered resigning from SAGE.

The newly opened economy, buoyed by such schemes as Eat Out to Help Out, was slowly feeding the virus. It still rankles with John Edmunds that taxpayers, including SAGE advisers, effectively subsidised the spread of the virus.

From July 2020 onwards, the infection rates began creeping up week by week. This was in the run-up to schools reopening in September, which we knew would provide fertile ground for community mixing and potentially lift R by 0.3 or 0.4. A change in seasons also has a small additional impact thanks to people moving indoors (although seasonality does not make that much difference, as shown in the fact that the pandemic spread rapidly in all kinds of climates).

During those holiday months of summer 2020, I felt very strongly that not enough had been done, particularly in terms of TTI, to prepare for the winter. In autumn, it was still too early to pin hopes on the vaccines but, then again, there was a misperception that the worst was behind us. At that point, we did not know about a new variant of coronavirus that would turn out to be more transmissible than the ancestral strain from Wuhan and prove harder to contain in the UK. Still, the older variant was sufficiently contagious to cause future waves of infection in a population that was still non-immune.

Everything from July onwards was heading in the wrong direction. And then, on 16 August, news leaked that Public Health England was going to be abolished. Even worse, Dido Harding, who had failed to establish the world-beating TTI system promised over the summer, was appointed interim executive chair of PHE's replacement, the National Institute for Health Protection. I just could not believe that Public Health England (PHE) was being thrown under the bus in the middle of a pandemic while the figurehead responsible for the TTI system was being promoted.

PHE was, in effect, being blamed for the coronavirus crisis, which at best was passing the buck. At the very least, it was disingenuous. While PHE lacked testing capacity in January, February and March of 2020, its impotence was the consequence of neglect over at least a decade. There were some very good people working desperately hard there during the pandemic, at both the local and national level, but austerity starved PHE of the funding it needed to handle a crisis of this magnitude. This was absolutely not the time to rubbish an agency that the country would need to call on as winter approached. I made public my displeasure, tweeting:

Arbitrary sackings. Passing of blame. Ill thought through, short term, reactive reforms. Out of context of under investment for years. Response to singular crisis without strategic vision needed for range [of] future challenges. Pre-empting inevitable public enquiry.

A junior UK minister in the Department of Health and Social Care complained about my tweet to Eliza Manningham-Buller, chair of Wellcome. Weeks later, the government announced it was considering Operation Moonshot, a plan to roll out rapid mass testing nationwide in a bid to keep the economy open. It would reportedly cost in the region of £100 billion. The *British Medical Journal* noted that the enormous sum was within touching distance of the entire annual budget for the NHS in England. Professors of public health, meanwhile, were telling the government that the tests under consideration were nowhere near foolproof, with substantial risks of both false negatives and false positives.

On 13 September 2020, I let rip about my frustrations to a handful of Wellcome colleagues in an update:

June–August was not used well enough to put in place what was needed, too much optimism that the worst was over and it could not be so bad again, continued focus on short term tactics, defending the indefensible, confirmation bias, and the lack of any central leadership or strategy ... Time has been wasted with distractions of 'moonshots', blaming the young or travellers/borders, the public enquiry, getting rid of PHE damaging morale of the very people who will be needed over the [next] 6 months, not preparing the NHS, TTI is very close to collapse at the moment...

If it can be prevented what needs to happen? (What should have happened June–August)

Get the 'boring' basics right and ready for autumn/winter, implementing what we know works and just do it well

Value competence above rhetoric

Be honest and transparent about the situation and what is needed

Narrow the gap between the advice, what we know needs to happen and the capacity to implement it

Strengthen the Cabinet Office, No 10, or a new grouping to oversee this, not driven by political announcements but by making a real difference

Does this need a cross party, national emergency crisis approach?

Admit not everything is working, conduct an immediate review, within a week reset a real, joined up strategy...

Stop trying to pretend 'it's all world beating' – it is not and everyone knows it, repeating that only loses more trust...

Later in the update, I asked my colleagues to think deeply about how close the Wellcome Trust should remain to the government, given the ongoing poor decision-making. The UK was heading into autumn having squandered the summer; NHS staff were shattered; PHE staff were demoralised, with some about to be fired; the education sector and local authorities were fighting their own battles with central government, particularly over safety in schools; it felt as if the public had lost trust in central government.

'By remaining in central advisory roles,' I asked, genuinely reaching out to my colleagues in a mood of deep despair, 'are we complicit in the outcomes?'

As I was agonising in mid-September over the prospect of damage by association, one of the deadliest decisions in the UK's handling of the pandemic lay just over a week away.

❋ ❋ ❋

SAGE met, via Zoom, on Monday 21 September 2020. The rise in transmission over the summer was clearly revealing itself, with the incidence of Covid-19 shooting up in all age groups. Infections seemed to be doubling every week, and this was before the full impact of school reopening had soaked in. Hospitalisations were rising, as were intensive care admissions.

The advice from that SAGE meeting was unambiguous: 'A package of interventions will be needed to reverse this exponential rise in cases...' The measures included a 'circuit breaker', or a short lockdown; advice to work from home; banning the mixing of households, except those in support bubbles; closing cafés, bars, restaurants, indoor gyms and personal services, such as hairdressers; and moving university and college learning online.

An accompanying paper summarising the impact of various measures noted that 'not acting now to reduce cases will result in a very large epidemic with catastrophic consequences in terms of direct COVID related deaths and the ability of the health service to meet needs'. The burden of a large second wave would 'fall disproportionately on the frailest in our society, but also those on lower incomes and BAME [Black, Asian and minority] communities'.

Faster, more stringent restrictions would mean fewer Covid-19 deaths, the minutes spelled out, and measures were needed both locally and nationally, rather than being tied to narrow geographical areas. That evening, Patrick and Chris gave a televised press conference warning there could be 50,000 new cases and 200 deaths a day by November if nothing changed. Notably, there were no ministers at that briefing.

Dominic Cummings has shed disturbing new light on the events in September 2020 and the efforts made to persuade Johnson that a circuit breaker was needed. By that time, Cummings said, there was unanimity among Patrick, Chris, Ben Warner and John Edmunds that intervention was needed. The Prime Minister did not want to act.

Cummings claims that, in order to try to change Johnson's mind, he organised a meeting on Tuesday 22 September 2020, at which Johnson was presented with the case numbers and infections rates by Catherine Cutts, a data scientist newly recruited to Number 10. She showed Johnson the current data and then fast-forwarded a month, to role-play the scenario of infections and deaths projected for October. Cummings says: 'We presented it all as if we were about six weeks in the future. This was my best attempt to get people to actually see sense and realise that it would be better for the economy as well as for health to get on top of it fast. Johnson basically said, "I'm not doing it. It's politically impossible and lockdowns don't work.'"

Johnson reportedly told Cummings that he should never have locked down in the first place and that he felt Cummings had manipulated SAGE into calling for the March lockdown. This allegation that SAGE was 'manipulated' is untrue.

Cummings says: 'Six weeks later on 31 October, we had pretty much exactly the meeting that we had predicted on 22 September would happen. If we didn't lock down immediately.' Cummings asserts that everyone in Number 10 knew that Johnson would end up locking down when it became clear there was no alternative.

Whatever happened behind the doors of Number 10, the government chose not to act in September 2020. Or, rather, it chose to not impose a lockdown – only a 10pm curfew and a request for people to work from home. I respect the mantra that scientists advise and ministers must decide, but ministers were clearly overriding SAGE advice, often while claiming to follow it.

Not acting is a decision in itself – and it had awful consequences. This was not March 2020, where, if you were exceptionally charitable, you could just about claim that we did not know the epidemic was coming and the data was poor. Back in March 2020, ministers could, at a stretch, have said they did not want to make a decision as grave as locking down the country on the basis of infectious disease modelling and the possibly overblown fears of public health doctors. That's not what I believed, but you could just about rationalise the late lockdown in March in that way.

Six months later, in September 2020, the government had no such excuse. We had already been through it. We knew what a lockdown could achieve – and the terrible impact of delaying it. There was no way that the lack of action could be blamed on poor data: by the autumn of 2020, the UK were collecting some of the best epidemiological data in the world. And that data was clearly showing the epidemic was climbing, week after week after week. R was above 1 (at the next SAGE meeting, on 24 September, it was recorded in the minutes as lying between 1.2 and 1.5).

Thanks to the rear-view mirror effect, we also knew that the number of deaths reported on the day of that 21 September SAGE meeting – 11 – reflected the state of the epidemic three to four weeks previously. That day also saw more than 4,000 new infections reported: over three to four weeks, some of those infections would turn into illnesses, illnesses would turn into hospitalisations and, sadly, some hospitalisations would turn into deaths. As the government remained rooted to the spot, transmission was already getting away from us. It was a catastrophe playing out in slow motion.

That was the darkest moment of the pandemic. I began to question the point of giving advice to a body that chose not to use it. There comes a time when you have to ask yourself, and the people you trust, whether you are indeed complicit with the decisions that are made as a result.

And then you wonder what will happen if you resign. Will it make any difference? You might feel better for an hour; it might generate headlines for a day, maybe two. The pandemic will still be there, except worse. And the world will move on. Eventually, you arrive at the somewhat arrogant conclusion that the system is probably better for your advice feeding into it.

That was the opinion of Eliza Manningham-Buller, the former intelligence chief who chairs the Wellcome Trust and who was privy to my confidential updates. Having found herself in similar situations as a government adviser, she believed that, when things got difficult, it was better to remain inside the tent. She thought it best I stayed to make sure reasonable scientific advice was still being heard, even if ignored. I texted Patrick, too: his view was the same.

Apart from Neil Ferguson, who really had no option but to resign from SAGE after bending lockdown rules, no other SAGE advisers have resigned. That is thanks to Patrick and Chris's leadership: they encouraged everyone to talk freely and frankly about their view of the science and the data, as long as it did not breach national security or stray into operational matters. They have done well to keep SAGE together for so long. Still, I would be very surprised if other SAGE advisers didn't at some point think, 'Why am I doing this?'

I wonder whether Chris or Patrick also occasionally thought of walking away from it all, though I have never asked them. I would be extremely surprised if they hadn't.

It is sobering to look back at historical eras in public health when terrible things happened. The scientists and doctors certainly do not come out of it well, and often deserve not to. Which brings me back to the central moral dilemma: does staying in an advisory role mean being complicit in the outcomes of bad decisions? To be honest, I still don't know the answer.

❄ ❄ ❄

On 14 October, England was split into three tiers so that restrictions could be applied more regionally rather than across entire nations. Tier 1 would enjoy the loosest restrictions; and Tier 3 the strictest, almost a lockdown. I understood the reasoning behind it – national shutdowns can be a blunt tool – but it did not bode well that its complexities had to be carefully explained with every airing. Tiers differed in their rules on indoor and outdoor gatherings, household mixing, dining out, worship, exercise and travel. Any system that requires the person explaining it to constantly look at their notes while spelling it out to the public is going to be a problem.

Britain is also a small, dense and highly connected island, with people travelling in and out of cities on a daily basis to work or see family and friends. The borders between tiers were arbitrary and permeable, and there was pretty much free flow across them anyway. It seemed fanciful to imagine we could exert enough precision of control over the epidemic to contain rises within regions. Some of us felt at the time that Tier 3 was not enough to control the epidemic, which simply meant higher tiers would seed the lower tiers and eventually, with all the laces tightened, the entire country would end up in the same straitjacket.

By the autumn of 2020, the UK was world-beating at something: gathering national data on coronavirus infections. Back in March 2020, I had teamed up with Ian Diamond of the Office for National Statistics to chair a meeting that led to the ONS infection survey, a random sampling of the population. In addition to the ONS study, Imperial College London and the polling company Ipsos MORI launched the REACT (Real-time Assessment of Community Transmission) study in April 2020. The REACT study has two arms: one counts how many people are currently infected, and the other tallies how many people have developed antibodies (and therefore have been infected in the past). The VIVALDI study, led by the brilliant Laura Shallcross at University College London, looks at the same two metrics – current infections and past infections – specifically in care homes.

Every Thursday evening, a bunch of us – including Ian, Laura and Paul Elliott, and Steven Riley from Imperial – have a 'data call', which is just a run-through of how the data looks and whether it is trending in any particular direction. We sometimes look at the information gathered by the ZOE Covid Symptom Study, led by Tim Spector at Kings College in London, so we can triangulate with other data to see if trends are consistent, or investigate why they are not. We are usually joined by Jeff Barrett, from the Wellcome Sanger Institute in Cambridge; the institute helps to carry out genomic sequencing that allows us to keep an eye on variants.

The meetings are co-chaired by Martin Innes at the Department of Health and Social Care (DHSC). Martin heads the Covid-19 Data Surveillance Strategy for the department and collates and circulates what is known as Pillar 4 data. This is national surveillance data that gives a current picture of how the epidemic is running.

On Thursday 22 October 2020, we waded through the usual tranche of data and Martin sent his summary. The data was as dismal as expected: the tiers were not holding back the tide. More than 20,000 new infections were being reported each day. This was exactly a month after SAGE had advised the circuit breaker package of interventions to stop transmissions.

As usual, Martin sent his summary and solicited comments from the 30-plus people on that Covid-19 data email list. I was certainly ready to oblige and hit 'reply all', meaning my blunt take would be seen by senior figures from Public Health England and the DHSC:

Thanks Martin

Does this summary make crystal clear that the data is unequivocal, consistent, has been since mid-July, predictable and very very worrying.

We are watching an epidemic unfold in front of us and simply spread from local to regional to national, slower than in

February and March ... but on a clear path to a winter disaster. It feels like we are sleep walking towards it, but worse, because we can see it, document it, we are watching the data unfold in front of us. And worse than sleep walking because it is so obvious, and because we have been here before.

Every so often we grasp what we think is a chink of light, a minor downturn in one region, in one piece of data and think we are turning a corner. We are not. That is confirmation bias at its worst. We are ignoring the elephant in the room – all ages, all regions, are increasing, the tiers are not effective ... and we are watching tier one become tier 2, tier 2 becoming tier 3 and tier 3 getting worse. We are also seeing worrying signs of increasing hospital transmission and of infections in the care home sector.

This is the most worrying period since the 10–23rd March....

We cannot continue to just watch it, delay decisions, or hope for the best and keep our fingers crossed.

I am not sure if others share my concerns – but I found the Pillar 4 data review today, the latest ONS and React data and then SAGE profoundly depressing and a major concern.

Jeremy

✳ ✳ ✳

The SAGE meeting on 22 October was similarly unequivocal. The minutes laid out the signposts towards that winter disaster: an epidemic growing exponentially; an R of between 1.2 and 1.4; modelling that was showing between 53,000 and 90,000 new infections a day in England. Surveys suggested an average of 433,000 people were, at that moment, infected just in England.

The associated deaths, some which could have been averted by a September lockdown, were already baked in, the minutes noted: 'Even if significant interventions sufficient enough to bring R below 1 were imposed immediately, the number of deaths would continue to rise...' There were markers of rising infections in care homes and university halls of residence, but, thanks to the rear-view mirror effect, those outbreaks had inevitably grown since.

All the numbers vindicated what Patrick and Chris had been saying publicly, and privately to Number 10, for a month: that things needed to change or the UK could see 200 deaths a day and 50,000 new infections a day by November. They were derided at the time for scaremongering. As November approached, Patrick and Chris saw their nightmares materialising. On 27 October, 367 Covid-19 deaths were confirmed (defined as a death within 28 days of a positive Covid-19 test). On 12 November, the number of daily confirmed new infections spiked at more than 33,000; the true number was closer to 95,000.

※ ※ ※

If scientists were advocating a lockdown, many politicians definitely were not. On 4 November, I was invited to talk via Zoom to the Covid Recovery Group, a group of 80 or so Conservative MPs in the UK Parliament. (I briefed the Shadow Cabinet on another occasion). I explained why tight restrictions were needed, highlighting rises in infections, hospitalisations and deaths. They asked questions like, 'What should I say to my constituents who don't see much Covid?'

I kept coming back to the point that you can either act now for a shorter time or you can act later for longer. You have a choice, but only when it comes to timing: you cannot choose whether to act or not. That is exactly the message that I have been giving to Emmanuel Macron from late 2020. We cannot begin to comprehend the anguish of a leader who is deciding whether to shut down his or her country, but the later the action, the more lives that will be lost and the more disruption to all sectors of society: schools, businesses, leisure, transport. Governments are eventually forced to act because they cannot simply stand by and watch their health systems collapse, as happened in the UK in March 2020.

The MPs listened respectfully and, in a passive-aggressive sort of way, were apparently thankful for me appearing before them. But did I change anyone's mind? No. Their minds seemed already made up and I believe the majority went on to vote against restrictions.

I have thought deeply about why my scientific world view was anathema to those MPs. One reason is ideology: libertarianism is one of their guiding principles. Lockdowns are a sign of big government and undoubtedly curb individual freedoms in a draconian way that none of us want. But the alternative is worse, as we have discovered.

Another hurdle I faced was that other scientists were offering different opinions. By early October, the Great Barrington Declaration* was getting a lot of publicity as an 'alternative' scientific theory. This was the dangerous proposition to allow the virus to sweep through the population quickly so that herd immunity could build up. The three professors who were pushing it – Jay Bhattacharya from Stanford University, Sunetra Gupta from Oxford University and Martin Kulldorff from Harvard University – essentially repackaged the herd immunity concept as 'focused protection'. Its proponents had been invited to present their thinking to Number 10 the previous month, a

---

* The Great Barrington Declaration was launched on 4 October 2020 at the American Institute for Economic Research, a free market thinktank in Great Barrington, Massachusetts.

meeting thought to have influenced Johnson's decision not to heed SAGE's advice to lock down.

The Great Barrington Declaration was ideology masquerading as science and the science was still nonsense. There was no evidence to support its central idea that herd immunity was a viable strategy. Earlier in the year, one of its scientists, Sunetra Gupta, had claimed that half of the UK had already been infected and therefore the UK was on its way to acquiring herd immunity.

The antibody data showed nothing of the sort; only 6 per cent of the UK population had been infected by September 2020, nine months into the epidemic. At that point, the Declaration believers explained away the discrepancy between their theory and the antibody data by suggesting people were protected by 'immunological dark matter'. It was an evidence-free assertion, as was the insistence by the Great Barringon supporters that there would be no second wave.

Dominic Cummings claims he had wanted to run an aggressive press campaign against those behind the Great Barrington Declaration and to others opposed to blanket Covid-19 restrictions, such as Carl Heneghan (an Oxford University professor and GP), the oncologist Karol Sikora and *Mail on Sunday* columnist Peter Hitchens.

Cummings says: 'In July, I said to [Johnson], 'Look, much of the media is insane, you've got all of these people running around saying there can't be a second wave, lock-downs don't work, and all this bullshit. Number 10's got to be far more aggressive with these people and expose their arguments, and explain that some of the nonsense being peddled should not be treated as equivalent to serious scientists. They were being picked up by pundits and people like Chris Evans [the *Telegraph* editor] and Bonkers Hitchens [Peter Hitchens].'

According to Cummings, Johnson rejected the idea of being more aggressive with the media, saying, 'The trouble is, Dom, I'm with Bonkers. My heart is with Bonkers, I don't believe in any of this, it's all bullshit. I wish I'd been the Mayor in *Jaws* and kept the beaches open.'

Herd immunity by natural infection was, and still is, a coronavirus strategy that lacks credibility. I cannot even call it science. Nonetheless, conflicting expert opinions serve a useful purpose, as they do in climate research: they allow politicians and others, sometimes even scientists themselves, to pick a world view that suits a pre-existing ideological bias.

On top of that, it has proved hard, regrettably, for some politicians to grasp that our view of an epidemic is always in the past. That, again, can bolster an ideological position if you are unwilling to understand the rear-view mirror effect. If you are against lockdowns, then you could look at 21 September, when there were eleven reported deaths, and say, 'Well, we're a country of 60 million people and we're not going to be frightened of a disease causing eleven deaths a day. The epidemic came to an end in June and we don't think it's coming back.'

For the record, nobody is *pro*-lockdown. Lockdowns are a last resort, a sign of failure to control the epidemic in other ways. Locking down does not change the fundamentals of a virus but buys time to increase hospital capacity, testing, contact tracing, vaccines and therapeutics.

Those behind the declaration, who managed to recruit people running the country to their cause, have done a great disservice to science and public health (that is the price one pays for the principle of academic freedom). There was no data to support their theory, as immunology studies bear out. Danny Altmann, professor of immunology at Imperial

College in London, described the central tenet of the Great Barrington Declaration as 'nonsense', and added that he could not see immunologists among the signatories. 'It was unfortunate that their views could command such attention,' Danny says.

Nonetheless, they got a lot of airtime and had the ear of those in government, particularly in the US and UK, who shared the same optimism bias for an easy solution. Frankly, I think their views and the credence given to them by Johnson were responsible for a number of unnecessary deaths.

❋ ❋ ❋

On 28 October 2020, Emmanuel Macron put France into another lockdown. I had been corresponding with a member of the Joint Biosecurity Centre, who by then had been to-ing and fro-ing for five days with several experts, including me, asking for more graphs and data analysis to feed into policy decisions.

Earlier, on 23 October, I had vented my desperation to him:

I know how unpalatable this is, but now, I do not see any alternative to a national lockdown – we are gradually edging towards it anyway, but by edging towards, with all the associated confusion, you will have to have it in place longer ... But UKG has to act, the current incremental approach, piece meal, step by step and hoping something turns around is not working. We are slipping into a winter nightmare.

By 28 October, I felt the government either did not know, or did not want to reveal, what its policy objectives truly were. It looked to me as if the (misguided) purpose of not instigating lockdown was to save the economy at the cost of lives and health.

That required being straight with the public. I emailed my Joint Biosecurity Centre contact again (he must have looked forward to opening my missives):

We are currently on track for 1000 deaths/day by end November if we do not change approach soon. Even if we do tragically many of those people are now in the system.

Every day now of delays in decisions are decisions in themselves with consequences. We are over a month since SAGE recommended the circuit break.

To be blunt. We locked down too late in March costing thousands of lives. We are making the same mistake again. But this time we knew, we have had the data, we know the disease better.

The current measures are caught in the middle. Will not change the path of the epidemic but are hurting the economy for little health benefit. The worst of all worlds.

These are rightly political decisions. But if the political decision is to accept 1000 deaths/day and the disruption of the NHS then the politicians need to explain that objective honestly to the public.

It took another week before the cogs of government whirred into action: a national lockdown finally came into force on 5 November 2020. The public were told it would be lifted on 2 December. While businesses need some degree of certainty to plan, we know from information that flows into the Joint Biosecurity Centre such as anonymised data from mobile phones, credit cards and transport networks – that people adjust their behaviour at the beginning and end of a lockdown. They take a while to settle into the restrictions, and then start relaxing about a week ahead of the official easing.

By announcing the dates of a one-month lockdown, the UK ended up with one that in reality lasted two to three weeks.

When lockdown was lifted on 2 December, R was still hovering around 1. The complexity of the tiering system became evident when hospitality venues in Tier 2 were informed they could serve alcohol with a 'substantial' meal. Much of the public debate that week was devoted to whether a scotch egg counted as a substantial meal. One food wholesaler saw demand for the hefty snack, a boiled, shelled egg encased in sausage meat and breadcrumbs, soar tenfold as pubs sought to cater (literally) to the restrictions.

By 19 December, after people had been mixing indoors and families were preparing to gather over Christmas (they had been told that three households could mingle for five days), transmission had risen sufficiently for the government to bolt on a fourth tier of restrictions. Rules for Christmas mixing were abandoned at the eleventh hour, as cases carried on increasing.

But another national lockdown did not come into force until 5 January 2021, just one day after some schools reopened. At that towering January peak of the second wave, Covid-19 deaths were exceeding 1,000 a day.

While a more transmissible variant of the virus made its debut in Kent in September, something we will explore in the next chapter, it worsened a disaster that was already brewing. The missteps are clear: the decision on 21 September 2020 not to introduce a circuit breaker; the wait until November before locking down; the premature lifting of lockdown on 2 December.

These set the scene for what can only be described as the carnage of January and February 2021. The loss of life in that short period dwarfed the first wave in spring

2020. 'Tragedy' is too mundane a word to describe what happened: many of these deaths were preventable.

As I told my Joint Biosecurity Centre contact back in October, the government seemed to be trading away the nation's health under the misguided belief it would protect wealth and the economy. I sent him a graph showing the link between the levels of transmission and the state of the economy for many industrialised nations.

The graph was split into quadrants, with the bulk of countries falling across a diagonal: at top left, countries with low transmission and relatively light economic disruption; at bottom right, countries with high transmission, like the UK, which had borne a dismal health toll and an economic kicking.

I added:

This [graphic] shows the relationship between controlling transmission and the economy. Countries that have achieved the former help the latter. With current measures we are heading further into the bottom right of this graph.

The UK strategy, such as it was, seemed doomed to economic and public health failure. The lessons from other countries in the first half of 2020 were that, in public health, trying to be too clever or trying to fudge it a bit does not work. You can throw the kitchen sink at public health, as New Zealand and Australia did, which kept rates in those countries to almost zero, but, otherwise, half-measures do not deliver even close to half the benefit. They are, literally, a false economy.

The UK was approaching the issue half-heartedly but paying double the penalty: people in the UK were dying in horrific numbers and the economy was tanking. By 23 March 2021, exactly a year after the UK entered its first lockdown, the death toll from Covid-19 stood at 126,172, much of which was racked up in 2021 – and the country had suffered its sharpest economic downturn for three hundred years.

8

The vaccines vs the variants

27 December 2020

Known global cases: 79,231,893
Global deaths: 1,754,574
UK cases: 2,256,009; UK deaths: 70,405
(within 28 days of a positive Covid-19 test)

AS 2020 PETERED OUT, the UK became a Janus: gazing at both failure and success at the same time.

The failure was rising transmission. As SAGE minutes noted on 17 December 2020: 'It is concerning that case rates are continuing to rise in areas that have been in Tier 3 ... Additional interventions may need to be considered in such places in order to keep R below 1 as per previous SAGE advice.' An extra tier came into force in the UK the week before Christmas 2020, vindicating advisers who had warned previously that the third tier would not be sufficient to hold the breach.

The success was the progress on vaccines: the UK became the first country to approve a fully tested Covid-19 vaccine (China and Russia approved home-grown vaccines before the final phase of trials had concluded). The approved vaccine, produced collaboratively between Pfizer and a German company called BioNTech, was a trailblazer for a new kind of jab using messenger RNA (or mRNA) technology. Whereas conventional vaccines are generally formulated using proteins from the pathogen, mRNA vaccines simply use the genetic code for the protein. This genetic code is piggy-backed into the body inside an envelope of lipids (proteins), where the body's own cells read the code and generate the corresponding protein. That newly produced protein then triggers the immune system to produce protective antibodies.

Messenger RNA vaccines essentially outsource protein manufacture to the human body, meaning they are potentially quicker to produce and quicker to adapt. The approval of the Pfizer–BioNTech vaccine, on 2 December 2020, came just seven months after clinical trials began.

The Oxford–Astra Zeneca (Ox–AZ) vaccine was approved four weeks later, at the end of December 2020. This was fantastic news: the Ox–AZ vaccine, which does not use mRNA technology, is being manufactured on a not-for-profit basis and can be stored in regular fridges rather than at ultra-cold temperatures, making it cheaper and easier to distribute (the Pfizer–BioNTech vaccine requires long-term storage at −70°C but can be kept for up to two weeks at around −20°C; in May 2021, the Food and Drug Administration in the US gave the go-ahead for the vaccine to be kept in a regular fridge for one month, to aid the roll-out).

The good news kept coming: in January 2021, the mRNA vaccine developed by Moderna became the third vaccine to win UK approval. It was just a year since I had sat alongside Moderna CEO Stéphane Bancel at Davos, where his compa-ny's CEPI-funded ambition to develop a coronavirus vaccine was announced.

Stéphane still remembers how emotional he felt when he took the phone call at home revealing the Moderna vaccine was 94 per cent effective, with Tony Fauci congratulating him: 'I remember leaving the call and going to my wife and crying. I was just thinking of all the people it would help. We have all seen the drama and turmoil and deaths, but also the side effects of a pandemic: the learning inequalities in children of low-income families, teens and young adults having their youth taken away and suffering mental health issues.

'And the older people, like my mum, who has blood cancer and has so little runway left. They have been locked down instead of travelling the world or seeing friends. All the people who lost their jobs, like the chefs I know whose businesses have gone under. After all that pain, the fact we could help people was such an amazing human feeling.'

Approvals elsewhere in the world, including the US and EU, soon followed for the mRNA vaccines. The regulatory passage of the Ox–AZ vaccine has been more painful, thanks to a combination of trial pauses due to adverse events, questions over study design and data analysis, and a link between the vaccine and a rare type of blood clot.*

If 2020 was an unremitting torrent of despair, 2021 suddenly seemed more hopeful. Science really was the exit strategy. Three effective vaccines anointed in quick succession energised the idea of vaccinating away the pandemic. Although it was unclear to what degree the vaccines could block infection and transmission, they were highly effective at stopping serious illness and death: Pfizer–BioNTech with

---

* The European Medicines Agency reports that about 1 in 100,000 people given the vaccine may suffer from an unusual blood clot that could be fatal in a minority of cases. In April 2021, the UK Joint Committee on Vaccination and Immunisation recommended that healthy under-40s be offered an alternative vaccine, although reiterated that the benefits of the vaccine outweigh the risks in all adults.

an efficacy of 95 per cent; Moderna with 94 per cent; and Ox–AZ with between 62 and 90 per cent, depending on how the data was sliced.

A year after the coronavirus surfaced, the pandemic exit plan swam into view: mass vaccination programmes across the world would be a precursor to unlocking economies and resuming normality. Countries like the UK already had a surfeit of the winning vaccines on order in tightly worded contracts: the UK's Vaccine Taskforce, for example, led by the redoubtable Kate Bingham, backed the science, sorted the supply chains, prepared the regulators and advance-purchased a total of 367 million doses of seven different vaccines – all before any final trial results were in. Experts were already gathering on the UK's Joint Committee on Vaccination and Immunisation to determine which citizens would be first in line for the jabs.

There was a chink of hope: could this really be the beginning of the end of the pandemic in the UK?

❋ ❋ ❋

In late November 2020, as those vaccines were galloping down the final regulatory straight, Tulio de Oliveira, a Brazil-born geneticist who heads a major coronavirus genome sequencing effort in South Africa, was trying to figure out why cases were surging in the Eastern Cape. He and his team at KRISP, the KwaZulu-Natal Research Innovation and Sequencing Platform, realised the surge was being fuelled by a new variant of coronavirus with a distinctive set of genetic mutations, including some in the spike protein.

Tulio named the variant 501Y.V2, after one key mutation, N501Y, that seemed to gift the variant its greater spreading power. A disease that spreads more easily is concerning, simply because more people are caught in the viral net: the more people the virus infects, the greater the number who will die or require hospitalisation.

The ballooning literature on coronavirus mutations held other nasty surprises on N501Y: a related mutation had been seen in mink in Denmark, where the disease appeared to be passing from farmed mink to farm workers and then back again (phenomena called spillover and spill-back respectively). Antibody treatments could not as readily neutralise variants with this new mutation.

The discovery was a body blow. Most of the vaccines, and certainly the high-profile ones, were built on mimicking the spike protein, something that had raised some concerns. If the spike protein was shape-shifting, as seemed to be the case in South Africa, the vaccines might not work quite as well as anticipated. At worst, they might not work at all.

Tulio, a member of the WHO Virus Evolution Working Group on SARS-CoV-2, called an urgent meeting of his colleagues; this was exactly the kind of change in the virus that the group had been watching out for. The working group numbers around 20 scientists from all over the world and includes Andrew Rambaut, the Edinburgh University scientist who helped to shepherd the original coronavirus genome sequence into the public domain in January 2020.

On Tulio's tip-off, Andrew began scouring UK samples for the N501Y mutation. Tulio recalls, 'A few days later, Andrew replied, saying, "Oh God, we looked up that mutation in our database and we found this big cluster".' The mutations seemed to be concentrated in samples coming from a region in south-east England.

Then serendipity intervened: in early December, Andrew was in a genomics meeting at PHE where specialists were puzzling over a large cluster of cases in Kent that was growing despite the November lockdown. Andrew remembers: 'It was one of those chance things. I just said, "Hang on a second, those look like the ones I've just been looking at with these mutations in them".' Further investigation, including modelling from Imperial College, revealed its relatively fast growth rate. That shows the value, Andrew says, of joined-up science: it was the linking of genomic surveillance to PHE's epidemiological tracking that pinned down the importance of this new faster-spreading variant.

It turned out that the citizens of Kent were not flouting the rules, as had been suspected, but were stricken with a variant estimated to be 50–70 per cent more transmissible than the ancestral virus circulating in early 2020. There are still conflicting opinions as to whether the variant causes more severe disease.

On 8 December 2020 at 6.31am GMT, Margaret Keenan was injected with the Pfizer–BioNTech vaccine, the first time a Covid-19 vaccine was administered anywhere in the world outside a clinical trial. A week later, both the UK and South Africa formally notified the WHO of the worrisome variants circulating in their countries. The variant that was first detected in the UK is termed B.1.1.7; the one first detected in South Africa, named 501Y.V2, is also known as B.1.351.* Despite the best efforts of scientists to keep geography and disease apart, to avoid stigmatising regions, they are often informally referred to as the UK variant and the South Africa variant.

As of spring 2021, there is another variant that keeps us awake at night: P.1, also called B.1.1.28, first detected in January 2021 in travellers from Brazil who were screened at

---

* On 31 May 2021, the WHO revealed a new variant naming scheme: B.1.1.7, also known as 501Y.V1, is now the Alpha variant; B.1.351, also known as 501Y.V2, is the Beta variant; P.1, also known as B.1.1.28 or 501Y.V3, is the Gamma variant; B.1.617.2 is the Delta variant.

an airport in Japan, and perhaps inevitably referred to as the Brazil variant. A variant that originated in India, B.1.617.2 is also causing huge concern, because it is spreading rapidly beyond India, including in the UK.

But why do we get new variants at all?

✻ ✻ ✻

SARS-CoV-2 is an RNA virus, which means its genetic material is composed of RNA (ribonucleic acid) rather than DNA (deoxyribonucleic acid), the stuff of life that characterises humans and other mammals. Many other pathogens, such as influenza, hepatitis C and Ebola, are RNA viruses.

When the virus enters the body, it hijacks cells and takes over their machinery to begin replicating. During the RNA copying process, random mistakes called mutations creep in.

Mutations are a bit like genetic typos; SARS-CoV-2 clocks up around one or two mutations per month on average. Very occasionally, through sheer luck (for the virus, not for humans), a mutation will confer some biological advantage, such as enhancing transmissibility or enabling the virus to partially or fully evade the immune system, perhaps by binding more tightly to receptors or producing higher viral loads in the nose and throat. These versions of the virus, which bear 'successful' mutations, can out-compete, or crowd out, less well-adapted variants, because of the survival advantage conferred by those mutations. This is 'survival of the fittest' in action.

In this sense, the pandemic coronavirus is a constantly evolving pathogen, giving rise to new forms of the virus that are variously referred to as variants or lineages. Most die out; some become dominant. It is possible that B.1.1.7 evolved in a patient with a lengthy infection, meaning the virus was able to persist and mutate for a long period before arriving at its current, extremely transmissible form.

In the end, the evolution of variants is a numbers game. Since every infected person is a crucible in which the virus can mutate, high infection rates raise the chances of a nasty new variant being cooked up. That is very probably why the variants of concern have been traced back to countries like the UK, South Africa and Brazil, which have had poorly controlled transmission coupled with good genomic sequencing. Scientists believe that, in the second waves of infection, the virus encountered survivors with some natural immunity gained during the first wave. This put added pressure on the virus to evolve, resulting in the variants we have today. We have yet to see a variant emerge in countries like New Zealand or South Korea, which have controlled their epidemics and kept transmission rates low.

Not all mutations, or variants in which they congregate, are a cause for concern; some mutations do not change the way the virus behaves. Variants meriting further investigation are first designated a 'variant of interest' (VOI) or 'variant under investigation'(VUI), with the most worrisome being escalated to a 'variant of concern' (VOC). The variants originating in the UK, South Africa, Brazil and India are all VOCs. Their survival advantages lie in transmissibility and 'immune escape': they spread more easily than other variants, and vaccines may not be as effective against some of the variants.

Vaccine efficacy against new variants is inferred by taking blood samples from people who have developed antibodies after natural Covid-19 infection or vaccination, and exposing the newer variants to these neutralising antibodies. The antibodies stimulated by older strains of the virus are only partially effective at neutralising the variant first identified in South Africa.

A variant was one of SAGE's concerns in the UK throughout 2020. After ministers shunned the idea of imposing restrictions, such as the circuit breaker, in September, transmission rose in the UK. The measures advised by SAGE to lower transmission were not implemented and the virus was able to take off. That encouraged, if that is the right word, the new variant, B.1.1.7, to appear and to spread. It has since become one of the country's most successful exports; it is now the dominant variant in Europe and the US, though early evidence suggests that B.1.617.2, first identified in India, is displacing it.

If you allow the quantity of virus to rise in a population, then this will come back to haunt you, first in lost lives and later in the appearance of variants that have the power to change the course of the pandemic. As I wrote to my Wellcome colleagues on 14 February 2021, as the UK emerged from the deadliest period of the pandemic:

Worth just noting – UK has seen ~50% of all deaths [so far] in the last 7 weeks and >35% of all hospital admissions. Sobering. A reminder what happens if you lose control of an epidemic, if you make the wrong decisions, or poor decisions coincide with events beyond your control – new variants!

I am not sure that I was correct to say that new variants were beyond our control. A decision to do nothing is still a decision. By not going into a lockdown in September 2020, the UK epidemic was left to continue its upward trajectory. The decision not to act fostered the conditions for the arrival and then the domination of these new variants, which had a dramatic impact on the pandemic.

Nobody should be surprised at what has happened since. That same month, in February 2021, genome sequencing revealed that some samples of the UK variant, B.1.1.7, had acquired the E484K mutation. This mutation, also seen in the variant first detected in South Africa, is known as an 'escape mutation' because it appears to give the virus some immunity against antibodies to the variant originating in China. Given the link between E484K and immune escape, this altered variant poses a threat to both natural immunity and the UK vaccination programme.

Later in that circular, I laid out the significance of the variants to my Wellcome colleagues, and said this would necessitate second-generation, even third-generation, vaccines:

Variants

These remain a huge concern and will define the course of the pandemic through 2021 and beyond

I frame it (simplistically) as two overlapping drivers

1: The virus evolving as it biologically adapts to humans through binding to the human receptor ... theoretically the virus has a long way to go from an evolutionary perspective

2: The virus evolving as 'immune pressure' increases through natural infection and now vaccination

These two drivers will influence evolution of the virus.

I do not think it is any coincidence that the new variants were all reported in Q4 2020 and not earlier. We can anticipate further and possibly faster evolution in 2021...

Wherever the virus is given a licence to circulate, there is the risk of further variants emerging. In March 2021, a new variant was detected, by Tulio and others, in three travellers stopped at an airport in Angola. This variant is, as of June 2021, the most mutated form of SARS-CoV-2 ever documented, with 31 mutations compared to the ancestral Wuhan virus (sometimes called the wild-type virus) first seen in December 2019. Among those 31 changes are 11 mutations in the spike protein of the coronavirus, again including E484K.

The three travellers picked up in Luanda came from Tanzania, where coronavirus has raged largely unchecked thanks to a leader in denial. John Magafuli, Tanzania's president, consistently denied that coronavirus was a threat to his country. An outlier among African nations, Tanzania stopped reporting coronavirus infections and deaths to the WHO in May 2020, and even refused an offer of vaccines from COVAX. Magafuli claimed that his countrymen enjoyed God's protection, despite senior churchmen urging Tanzanians to take the virus seriously.

Magafuli vanished from view in late February 2021; an announcement came on 17 March that he had died. There is speculation that the 61-year-old president, who was fitted with a pacemaker for heart problems, succumbed to Covid-19. If so, he joins a throng of parliamentarians in Tanzania to have died after reportedly suffering Covid-like symptoms.

Covid denialism can be lethal.

※　※　※

'It's a shocker', says Sharon Peacock, of the new variant traced back to Tanzania. Sharon is professor of microbiology at Cambridge University, an expert in the genome sequencing of pathogens, and a fellow adviser on SAGE, the UK scientific collective that advises ministers. She is coming to the end of a two-year secondment to Public Health England.

Scientists in the UK have been at the forefront of looking out for variants, and none more diligently than Sharon, who was director of the National Infection Service at PHE at the beginning of the pandemic and has since become its director of science. Sharon had the vision to step sideways from PHE in order to quickly set up COG-UK, the Covid-19 Genomics UK Consortium, which has been steadfastly sequencing coronavirus samples in the country since April 2020. I am proud to say the consortium had its first meeting at the Wellcome Trust, where Sharon had been advising us on the globally important issue of antimicrobial resistance.

The wheels of COG-UK started turning on 4 March 2020, when Sharon sent a one-line email to five close contacts: Cambridge colleague Julian Parkhill, a former head of Pathogen Genomics at the Wellcome Trust Sanger Institute (dedicated to genome sequencing); Judith Breuer, a virologist at University College London; Nick Loman, an expert in microbial genomics and bioinformatics at Birmingham University; David Aanensen, a genomic surveillance specialist at the Big Data Institute at Oxford University; and Richard Myers, at Public Health England.

I wonder if you could call me on my mobile this afternoon, 2pm onwards. Sharon

By then, Sharon had joined SAGE and was being bombarded, as we all were, with hundreds of emails a day. Sharon remembers: 'I just wanted to cut through everything and get rapid feedback from colleagues I trusted. When they rang, I just said, "I think we need a national genome sequencing capability [on the coronavirus] and do you agree? If so, will you come to meeting about it next week?" It was like a rolling stone: getting five people gave me the confidence to ask 20 more people, and then it was a matter of grabbing everyone who was available.' Further invitees included Oliver Pybus, an expert in pandemic genomics at Oxford University and Emma Thomson, a specialist in infectious diseases at the Centre for Virus Research at Glasgow University.

Sharon borrowed a meeting room at the Wellcome's central London headquarters and, on 11 March, chaired the inaugural no-frills meeting of what would turn out to become COG-UK: 8.30am start, no sandwiches or refreshments (though we do have a very nice in-house café), a series of invitation-only 'lightning talks: max 5 minutes, max 2 slides'. I popped in at the beginning, just to welcome everyone.

Sharon's meeting wasn't about the science of genome sequencing; the UK was already a world leader in that. It was about getting a sequencing pipeline up and running operationally: feeding it coronavirus samples taken from all over the country through multiple agencies, such as PHE, NHS and TTI, processing the information at pace and using it to bend the epidemic curve.

'It was basically twenty of us shut in a room and we didn't leave until we had worked out the blueprint for how we'd do it,' she says now. The blueprint was on Patrick Vallance's desk by 15 March; two weeks later COG-UK banked £20m, ready to start work. I remember being in a taxi on the way to a SAGE meeting, talking on the phone to Mike Stratton, director of the Wellcome Trust Sanger Institute, negotiating how much the institute would put in.

Sharon's sense of urgency was well placed: between that initial 11 March 2020 meeting and the 1 April kick-off, confirmed coronavirus infections in the UK rose from about 1,300 to nearly 44,000.

Despite Patrick's fulsome support, the consortium had its detractors: SARS-CoV-2 does not mutate as quickly as influenza or HIV. 'There was quite a lot of criticism that COG-UK was an expensive stamp-collecting exercise,' Sharon recalls. 'People would tweet and challenge us, saying we were just sequencing the same virus over and over again, questioning whether it was a good use of public money. I had sleepless nights about it, thinking "What if all this sequencing is for nothing?" And I really struggled with people challenging me and saying, "Who gave you the right to go off and set up COG-UK?" To which I would reply, "Humanity, actually".'

Sharon comforted herself with the idea that, at worst, the consortium would produce a pile of interesting scientific papers; at best, the national sequencing programme meant the country would be ready for when the virus started acting up. Besides, she had the best virologists in the country backing her up, volunteering their services because they shared her belief that genome sequencing could help to keep tabs on an unpredictable virus. That the virus would mutate, she says, was never in doubt; the only unknowns were the timetable and the exact nature of the mutations.

Thankfully, Sharon kept the faith: 'That meeting at Wellcome with like-minded people gave me a real sense of optimism that we could pull this off. I just thought, I'm going to run with it. I'm going to make sure that we're ready for when the virus starts to evolve in a way that might worry us.'

By late 2020, the sleepless nights had stopped. COG-UK was no stamp-collecting exercise. The UK samples being processed through the pipeline that the consortium assembled were flashing hints of the new variants, dovetailing with Tulio's tip-off that the virus appeared to be changing significantly. COG-UK played a key role in unravelling the frequency and spread of B.1.1.7.

Now, the challenge is to vanquish existent variants and put the stopper back in the viral bottle by getting infection rates down. As Sharon says: 'Our ability to fight the variants will be in direct proportion to how far we can reduce infections in this country and around the world, because that's the key lever that we have in getting mutation rates down. It's about how quickly the vaccine can be rolled out and whether we can persuade people to continue behaviours like social distancing and hand-washing, rather than just going back to normal. And it will also depend on what we do about borders.'

Sharon has been concerned about the variant first detected in South Africa, B.1.351: 'That's the variant that seems to have the biggest hit in terms of vaccine escape. It's not full vaccine escape but it's quite significant and, in my view, that's the one that's going to be the first threat to our vaccine efficacy. If we can't get ahead of the variants, we will have a big problem on our hands.' A May 2021 paper in the *New England Journal of Medicine* suggests the Ox–AZ vaccine does not protect against mild-to-moderate illness caused by the B.1.351 variant; other studies suggest it prevents severe illness, hospitalisation and death across a range of variants, including B.1.351.

Since then, the B.1.617.2 (Delta) variant has burst on to the scene, first in India and now spreading worldwide. As of June 2021, it is displacing other variants in the UK; scientists are trying to assess whether it is more transmissible, causes more severe disease or is better able to evade vaccine-induced immunity. The UK government has faced criticism for not closing its borders to India sooner. The UK had been seeded with the Delta variant by returning travellers.

Tulio, though, is scathing about the idea of the UK closing its borders to keep variants out. He points out that there are already thousands of people in the UK infected with other variants containing similar mutations to those seen in B.1.351, meaning these other variants may pose a comparable threat: 'Closing borders helps islands like New Zealand [which has very few cases], not the UK. The UK government has done an appalling job of managing the epidemic and would do much better trying to control their own variants that have mutations of concern rather than scapegoating other countries.'

Long-term, he favours elimination, as countries like New Zealand, Australia and Taiwan have aimed for, with swift action to stop small outbreaks growing into bigger epidemics, which risk churning out further new variants. Elimination, he believes, would be less painful than running to keep up with variants and vaccinating the world every year. 'Don't treat it like the flu,' Tulio cautions. 'Treat it like a much more transmissible virus. The best solution is to almost eliminate transmission.'

I think eradication – ridding the world of the virus, as was done for smallpox – is impossible but that elimination – banishing the virus from countries or regions through control measures – is possible and indeed desirable. The virus is now endemic, which means it will continue to circulate globally for years to come, possibly for ever. The way forward is to reduce transmission to the lowest possible level through public health measures plus vaccination. Countries whose populations are comprehensively vaccinated can then aim for elimination .

❋ ❋ ❋

It is striking that the same mutations crop up again and again in lineages of the coronavirus in different countries, albeit in slightly different constellations. For example, the mutation in the spike protein known as E484K, seen in variant B.1.351 originating in South Africa, has appeared in some samples of the UK variant B.1.1.7. The 681H mutation seen in B.1.1.7, also in the spike protein and associated with increased transmissibility, has been clocked in the variant recently detected in Tanzania.

P.1, the variant originating in Brazil, and B.1.351 share a triplet of mutations: E484K, N501Y and K417N/T. A variant, B.1.617.2 linked to a spike in cases in India in April 2021, shares a mutation called L452R with a variant linked to a surge in California earlier the same year. These genetic encores, which have arisen independently in different parts of the world where the virus circulates, suggest the mutations give the virus a competitive edge over circulating variants.

As Tulio explains, there looks to be an apparent convergence in the way the virus is changing: 'We have convergent evolution. A lot of these variants have E484K, which affects neutralisation.' In other words, variants with E484K mutation appear able to sidestep neutralising antibodies, at least in the laboratory. This means that a person who has been infected with an older variant of coronavirus, or who has been given a vaccine designed around the spike protein of an old variant, might be susceptible to infection or reinfection by a new variant containing E484K. The mutated virus is sufficiently different from older variants that the immune system no longer wholly recognises it. South Africa is no longer using the Ox–AZ vaccine, because of worries about reduced efficacy against B.1.351. The India-linked variant contains E484Q, a related mutation that also enhances its ability to infect cells.

While vaccines are being updated – Moderna expects to have its booster ready by autumn 2021 – the big question is what the virus will do next. Is convergence the first step to settling down into a stable configuration? Even with two decades of experience in watching viruses evolve, Tulio shies away from futurology: 'We can see this very strong convergence but the virus has surprised us a million times over the past year and a half, and I wouldn't like to predict if it's going to be stable.' His fear is that future waves of infection could bring another substantial jump in evolution or fitness, hence his support of elimination as a strategy.

It would take a bold and brave person, Sharon concurs, to second-guess the virus. The virus was already a competent human pathogen when it emerged, she explains, and a subsequent burst of evolution has given rise to new variants with similar properties in a different part of the world. The virus will be constantly changing to become the fittest version of itself whether that is through increased transmissibility or the ability to outwit naturally acquired or vaccine-induced immunity: 'The big question is: will there be another shift and how much will it threaten our vaccine programme?

'It is possible that we get a third wave where the virus is doing something really different, perhaps by being ultra-transmissible or ultra-immune, like the kind of step up we saw around October 2020. Are we going to see that again? To tell you the truth, I don't know.'

✹ ✹ ✹

Reducing transmission and cutting the amount of virus circulating is central to heading off the future threat from new variants. So is vaccinating the world. That latter strategy underpins COVAX, the bid to bring two billion doses of vaccines in 2021 to countries and populations that would otherwise be unable to access them.

But that looks unlikely to happen, because the world cannot manufacture at the pace currently needed and countries that do hold vaccines are not sharing them. Demand for vaccines massively exceeds supply: we have 7.7 billion people exposed to the virus at almost at the same time and that has never happened before. The shortage cannot be solved by money alone: if governments choose to bilaterally sign contracts and tie up access to vaccines, as the UK, US and EU have done, no amount of money in COVAX will bring access to vaccines.

The UK, for example, is an incredibly powerful position, having secured access to a total of 367 million doses made up of seven vaccines. That was necessary: no vaccine is guaranteed and the UK needed a wide portfolio to maximise the chances of success. We will now have substantial oversupply guaranteed by binding contracts, and the US is in exactly the same position. But much of the rest of the world has no ability to sign any contracts, because raw materials and manufacturing capacity (which is limited to less than a dozen countries) has already been taken up by countries that were able to pay early.

The bottleneck is exacerbated by countries changing their mind about who to vaccinate. Before the vaccines arrived, the UK envisaged vaccinating about 30 per cent of its population – basically healthcare workers and the over-50s. As the vaccines came on stream, that changed radically, partly because of the arrival of variants and fears of waning immunity and rising infection rates. Today, the plan is to vaccinate 100 per cent of the UK population, potentially including children if clinical trials show it is safe and effective. So, stocks that were earmarked for the vulnerable in other countries are being diverted into domestic supply.

The upshot is that we are now hoarding vaccines to immunise low-risk sections of the UK population while refusing to give up stocks to the rest of the world to stop people dying. One could pragmatically accept that a government's prime responsibility is to its own citizens, but we have ended up with an incredibly inequitable distribution of vaccines. I can see that it would be politically almost impossible for Boris Johnson or Matt Hancock to go out and say, 'Actually we're not going to vaccinate 30-year-olds anymore because we're giving our vaccines to Nigeria or Brazil. But it would be enlightened self-interest and the right thing to do. I just cannot see them doing it in time. And timing is key: leadership is not about getting to the right decisions eventually but reaching those decisions early. The arrival of the Delta variant (B.1.617.2) shows the importance of cutting transmission everywhere: nobody is safe until everyone is safe.

Instead, what has happened is an abrogation of international responsibility. I have probably said that at every single SAGE meeting in 2021 and I will carry on saying it until I am blue in the face. Patrick Vallance and Chris Whitty absolutely understand the need to vaccinate the world.

The spectre of vaccine nationalism has turned people like Tulio and me into vaccine activists: together with Tedros, we think vaccine apartheid is a fairer description of the current two-track pandemic. Tulio is horrified at the UK headlines generated by the very rare risk of blood clots in younger people linked to vaccination while healthcare workers in other countries are dying for want of a jab. This debate is also likely to be fuelling vaccine hesitancy in other countries.

To do better next time, we must solve the problem with vaccine supply. That means getting a wider range of countries involved. If vaccine manufacturing is confined to large countries or blocs like India, China, the US and Europe, then we will always run the risk of those countries reneging, in global emergencies, on contracts to supply other countries. In March 2021, India froze vaccine exports from the Serum Institute of India, a major contractor with COVAX, to deal with a worrying second wave in the country. I cannot blame India for doing this, as it is undergoing a horrific epidemic, but it means that other countries will have to wait longer for lifesaving interventions. John Nkengasong, director of the Africa Centers for Disease Control and Prevention, has identified this as an obstacle to vaccinating Africa.

The only solution I have come up with is that the world appoints maybe a dozen smaller-population countries to supply vaccines to the world. Countries could be paid by the global financial system, basically the World Bank and the International Monetary Fund, to do this; applicant countries could compete for 25-year contracts or leases. Countries would need to have populations lower than about 20 million, so that they could supply their own domestic populations immediately in an emergency and then start exporting very quickly after. I'm thinking of countries like Singapore, Norway, Denmark, Costa Rica, Senegal, Rwanda, New Zealand – they could become a global network of UN enterprise zones for manufacturing under a global mandate.

In the meantime, the UK and US could stake a claim to global leadership by drawing up a timetable for sharing surplus vaccine doses to which they are entitled under contract. These precious supplies should not be dispensed like last-minute giveaways, but according to a carefully planned schedule: it takes time to set up the cold chains, transport networks and labour force to deliver nationwide vaccine programmes.

Not to do so would be a failure of statecraft and diplomatic vision, threatening humanity's ability to build coalitions to address future pandemics, climate change, drug resistance and all the other global challenges heading our way. Stock-piling doses while other countries carry on counting their dead will lead many low- and middle-income countries to ask where the West was when they most needed help.

9

*This did not have to be a global pandemic**

30 MAY 2021

Known global cases: 169,604,858
Global deaths: 3,530,837
Vaccine doses administered (21 May): 1,448,242,899
UK cases: 4,480,949; UK deaths: 127,775

WHAT IF THE TAPE had run differently? What if those six miners who developed pneumonia after clearing droppings from bat caves in southern China[†] had been properly investigated? Imagine what could have happened if doctors had traced their infections back to a novel SARS-related coronavirus most commonly seen in bats. What if there had been a global system not only to pick that up, but also to raise an alert that humanity had no immunity against the virus, to immediately share virus samples globally with scientists and to trigger research into putative vaccines and treatments?

---

*   'This did not have to be a global pandemic.'Maria Van Kerkhove, WHO.
†   See p.74 for the background on this.

None of this is easy: it is a struggle to identify clusters and unmask a completely new pathogen at work. But, equally, none of it is beyond the capability of science.

✳ ✳ ✳

This is what we desperately need: surveillance in the shadowlands where humans and animals overlap, and specifically when those exchanges are leading to illness. We need to be asking: which viruses in wild and domestic animals are crossing back and forth between humans and animals? How can we spot these perilous cross-species breaches and how should we respond?

The pathogens that keep me awake at night are those against which humanity is defenceless. So, in the next five years, we need to document these gaps in the global human immune landscape. For a decade now, I have been wondering whether seasonal influenza, or winter flu, may not be the viral enemy we think it is, because the world has a degree of protection against many of the strains in the flu family.

Rather, the deadly black swan could be a radically different flu virus that reaches us directly from animals. It will contain proteins the human immune system have never encountered. Take H7N9 avian influenza, seen in poultry and other birds, and first detected in humans in 2013. There have been a handful of outbreaks since, mostly in China. Nearly 1,600 people have been infected in total, of whom more than 600 died. What if H7N9 suddenly acquired the ability to pass from person to person and was able to exploit that immunity gap? The consequences of a respiratory disease with a 30–40 per cent mortality rate that could transmit between people, possibly asymptomatically, does not bear thinking about. Even a mortality rate of 3–4 per cent would be apocalyptic.

Except that people *must* think about it. We are going through a period in human history, most obviously in the past twenty years, when global trends are aligning to cause more frequent and complex epidemics. Climate and ecological change, urbanisation, changes in food production and habitat loss are reshaping the way we interact with animals, boosting the chances of new diseases. When transmissible ones emerge, urbanisation and international travel accelerate their spread.

None of this is news to people like Marion Koopmans, from Erasmus University in the Netherlands, who sees the connection between disease and ecology (how people and animals relate to their environment) crop up again and again: 'If there's a big increase in animal density, if there is tearing down of forests for building, and if there is a shift in the food markets, that's when we see viral outbreaks.'

Marion worries that the interface between humans and other species, the Petri dish for new plagues, is a blind spot: 'We know that we are surrounded by all sorts of animal species that carry all sorts of viruses that we don't know about yet. Studies from the past two decades have taught us that if you go out and sample a group of animals, you will discover multiple new viruses. We don't know which of those viruses are a problem for humans.'

Many of the most serious disease outbreaks within living memory have been born at the human–animal interface: HIV-AIDS from chimpanzees; Ebola, SARS, MERS and Nipah from bats (sometimes via other species); H5N1 influenza from birds; Dengue, Chikungunya and Zika spread by mosquitoes. It is a pathogenic parade of relentless temporal regularity: Nipah in 1998, SARS in 2002, H5N1 in 2004, H1N1 in 2009, MERS in 2012, Ebola in 2013, Zika in 2015, Covid-19 in 2019. There are others besides.

Ebola is an example of what we might call twenty-first-century 'pathogen creep' – the phenomenon of pathogens exploiting the ecological niches we are carving out for them. From 1976 to 2014, the bat-borne virus only really terrorised small rural villages. Identifying an outbreak and closing off the village stopped the disease spreading. What changed in 2014, when the record outbreak in West Africa built up steam? The virus did not change but humanity did. People were moving more frequently between rural areas and urban centres, with cities amplifying outbreaks to cause massive disruption.*

So, what do we do, given that trends such as urbanisation, ecological change and climate shifts will define this century? On the positive front, there *is* action we can take. The prescription is clear and has been for many years: the world needs to pull together and treat pandemics as an existential threat to humanity. That means taking global health more seriously than it has ever been taken before, and planning for future pandemics (and the current HIV and tuberculosis pandemics) with the same gravity we accord to military security.

It needs a properly structured programme of science and research that scans threats in real time. It requires a muscular, independent World Health Organization to set public health standards, convene nations and to act immediately on the information that emerges. We need pipelines that can instantly produce tests, therapies, vaccines, oxygen and PPE. We should prepare a store of vaccine platforms against families of viruses, ready to plug the immunity gaps we discover and coupled with strategies for producing the

---

* Covid-19 has recalibrated what we regard as massive disruption. About 11,000 people died in that Ebola outbreak; I would guess there have been around 11 million Covid-19 deaths as of May 2021, several times the official tally.

vaccines in a hurry. There must be serious financing so that health systems all around the world are resilient enough to deal with a surge of disease when it strikes. The cost will be billions – but still only a fraction of the trillions the Covid-19 pandemic has cost so far.

It also requires a multilateral approach: countries must work together to reduce transmission for the good of all. Countries that eliminate Covid-19 – through a mix of border controls, vaccination and non-pharmaceutical measures such as quarantine and isolation – are still at risk (once they reopen) from new variants arising in other countries. Only the virus benefits from a pivot towards myopic nationalism, because that will keep it circulating for longer. A divided world is a diseased world.

※ ※ ※

Everything starts with smarter surveillance. If you don't look, you don't see. If you don't see, you will always respond too late. The UK government, in partnership with the Wellcome Trust, WHO, G7, EU and other organisations, is launching the Global Pandemic Radar (GPR). This will be a global surveillance system with a clear purpose: to identify clusters of disease; to prevent clusters seeding epidemics; and to prevent epidemics turning into pandemics.

It will unite traditional public health knowledge with twenty-first-century technology, such as genomic sequencing, the smarter use of data, artificial intelligence, plus non-traditional sources of information like rumours on social media. The blueprint for the Global Pandemic Radar is being finalised and, given there is no time to waste, should be functional this year. It will have the WHO at its centre, as it should, and has attracted input from people on every continent. It should close a gap that everyone in global health knows has existed for twenty years.

The GPR will be guided by a handful of fundamental principles. It should not reinvent the wheel but instead springboard from networks and structures already in place, such as the WHO flu surveillance network. It should have eyes on every continent, with regional hubs in cities like Lagos, Delhi, Beijing, Ho Chi Minh City, Moscow, Lima and Berlin, as well as in Atlanta and London. It should monitor for signs of antimicrobial resistance to drug treatments and endemic infections, as well as spotting new pathogens. Just as you do not wait until war has broken out to assemble and train an army, the radar must function continuously.

Critically, it must be able to trigger action in real time. Action means a public health response, like isolation and social distancing, plus diagnostics, drugs and vaccines.

❋ ❋ ❋

If the WHO has been perceived by some to be toothless, it is because the 194 member states who collectively decide what it does voted for it to be that way. (Contrary to those perceptions, the agency played a critical role in guiding countries, fast-tracking research, kick-starting clinical trials and setting up the ACT-Accelerator.) Each member sends delegates to the World Health Assembly, and it is the assembly which appoints the director general and decides what the WHO does.

The WHO did not police global health in the manner that many felt it should during the pandemic, because it was not designed or empowered to. Over time, the agency has been weakened, underfunded, undermined and politicised, a trend that climaxed with an event that none of us would have ever thought possible: the US pulling out of the WHO at the height of a pandemic.

The World Health Assembly now wants to change that sorry situation. In May 2020, the assembly commissioned an inquiry, *Covid-19: Make it the Last Pandemic*, led by Ellen Johnson Sirleaf, the former president of Liberia, and Helen Clark, the former prime minister of New Zealand. It examined the international health response and mused on the lessons to be learned to avoid such a crisis again.

The resulting report, published in May 2021, contained immediate recommendations aimed at ending the Covid-19 pandemic: increasing vaccine supply, including the waiving of patent rights on vaccines if needed, plus the continued use of measures like isolation, quarantine and social distancing to curb transmission.

As important are suggestions for how to make the WHO a stronger, more independent force for global health in the years to come. One idea is to introduce a single seven-year term for the WHO director general, rather than having shorter, renewable terms. This is something I support (though I would prefer eight years): a single term allows more independence from member states and frees the incumbent of having to seek re-election (as Tedros is doing now). Beefing up the WHO's autonomy and authority will allow it to release information on potential pandemic outbreaks without the approval of national governments. The report suggests increasing the budget of the WHO through hiking membership fees based on ability to pay and allowing the agency to spend it as it sees fit.

Its regional offices must be invested in. Patricia Garcia, the former health minister of Peru and a professor of global health in Lima, describes the contribution of the

Pan-American Health Organisation, the regional WHO office, to controlling Covid-19 in her country as 'peripheral'. That is heartbreaking, and a tragedy for the Americas, which have been particularly badly hit.

Significantly, the report suggests setting up a Global Health Threats Council, led by heads of state, and developing a pandemic treaty, putting pandemic preparedness and response on a similar legal footing to treaties covering climate change and human rights, which come within the purview of the United Nations. The report recommends an International Emergency Pandemic Financing Facility, controlled by this newly formed high-level council, able to immediately disburse up to $100 billion in the event of pandemic declaration using funds accrued through annual contributions. Any funding facility must be prepared to invest in global public goods with no obvious commercial incentive, such as a vaccine platform geared towards a virus that infected six miners.

Other recommendations include: each country having a national pandemic coordinator with a hotline to the top of government; and that the ACT-Accelerator, a pipeline set up in haste in 2020 that coordinates the scientific response from research to diagnostics, treatments and vaccines, is remoulded into a permanent fixture of the global health landscape. The Global Pandemic Radar is also part of the future strategy, and it will be essential for the global health community to think strategically about how best to simplify what we do.

※ ※ ※

My preference would be to streamline the architecture of global health: with the WHO in the middle of the web, convening, advising, guiding and providing an emergency response; an organisation like CEPI for research and development into countermeasures like diagnostic tests, treatments and vaccines, plus early manufacturing; an agency a bit like GAVI or Global Fund, or a merger of the two, that deals with procurement and delivery of the countermeasures; and a truly independent monitoring board that keeps an eye on progress, spots the gaps and speaks truth to power, whether to the UN Security Council or a new Global Health Threats Council.

Perhaps the biggest need is to radically overhaul the funding of global health. When we discuss global health, many people think it is about dreadful things befalling poor people in faraway places. The funding routes that spring to mind are aid and charity. We have organisations like GAVI and the Global Fund going hand to mouth to governments every few years, which results in a pledging conference. It is political theatre for presidents and prime ministers, and the result is crumbs from the table sprinkled sparsely across multiple agencies delivering essential work.

During the past fifteen months, I have attended these set-piece meetings, including at the World Health Assembly and the UN General Assembly, and found them intensely frustrating. Minister after minister gets up and reads out a pre-written statement. Frankly, they might as well be reading a bus timetable. If you listened to them all, you would think the world was in a great place, but what they say often bears almost no relationship to reality. They end up either talking past each other or weaponising health to score geopolitical points, as we have seen with the controversy over the origins of SARS-CoV-2.

Crumbs from the table will not cut it in an era of pandemics. What Covid-19 shows is that global health needs a bread basket. Protecting the health of our interconnected world insulates us all from the kind of mass disruption we are currently living through, some more painfully than others. For that reason, global health must be on the agenda of finance ministers and ultimately heads of states. Otherwise nothing will change. We need to put all the agencies that are working on global health and pandemic preparedness on a serious footing in the world financial order.

In my view, the pandemic has been a catastrophic failure of global diplomacy at just the time we need cooperation. The world is facing a deluge of transnational crises that cannot be navigated by individual countries alone: climate change; drug resistance; energy demand; water scarcity; conflict and migration. We must set new standards of global cooperation while recognising that the balance of power is shifting: from West to East; from North to South. There is a new world order, with a rising China, India, the African Union and the Americas (Patricia Garcia from Peru says she wants to see a Latin American Union modelled on the African Union). This should be acknowledged by organisations in which power resides: the G7, G20, World Bank, International Monetary Fund, United Nations and, of course, the World Health Organization. If we can find a way of tackling pandemics together, it will provide a blueprint for the other grave challenges that lie in store.

Gordon Brown, the former UK prime minister, is among many political figures who believe the status quo must change. He has taken a keen interest in how global public goods like global health are paid for, and how the financial system should be reformed to accommodate it. He has been vocal about vaccine inequality during the pandemic, and particularly in the run-up to the G7 meeting, held in June 2021 in the UK.

He wants to see increased funding for COVAX so that countries can immunise around 70 per cent of their populations (to reach herd immunity), rather than 20 per cent, as originally envisaged. That means raising around $60 billion to buy vaccines to make up the shortfall. 'The only sensible way of delivering something that is a life and death matter is not relying on pledging conferences or charity fundraisers but having a formula that people agree is based on fair shares based on capacity to pay and it being accepted by richest countries in the world,' Gordon says.

In essence, vaccinations would be paid for using a burden-sharing formula, with the richest countries paying the most, not only because they have the broadest shoulders but also because they will benefit most when trade and travel resume. A similar formula could be used to calculate contributions to strengthening basic healthcare in low- and middle-income countries, along with loans backed by guarantees from high-income countries. It is, Gordon believes, an insurance policy for the world. He also thinks the World Bank and regional development banks should play a greater role in public health, working through agencies like the WHO, GAVI, CEPI and Global Fund.

There is a precedent for splitting global bills: in 1967, a burden-sharing agreement was used to bankroll the WHO's smallpox eradication programme, which saw the disease stamped out across the world in 1980 (still the only human infectious disease that has been globally eradicated). Countries pay membership dues to UN organisations and services, such as UN Peacekeeping, on the basis of assessed contributions, which are similarly weighted on an afford-to-pay basis.

I hope the report from the World Health Assembly and the G7 and G20 reviews on this issue, which I have been involved with, will finally spur the change that has been needed for so long. We have had enough reviews. We have ticked too many of the same boxes in the past. We are past the time for action.

✹ ✹ ✹

One of the most striking outcomes of the pandemic is that the countries thought best prepared to face an outbreak of this magnitude were the US and the UK. While it is perhaps too early to pass final judgement on how they dealt with Covid-19, or indeed on how any countries have fared, these two wealthy nations have so far suffered comparatively high death rates.

The US and UK were ranked first and second, respectively, on the Global Health Security Index, assembled jointly by Sam Nunn's Nuclear Threat Initiative, Johns Hopkins University and the Economist Intelligence Unit. The index reflects a wide range of factors in each country that is thought to relate to ability to respond, including: disease surveillance; levels of immunisation; laboratory capacity; communications infrastructure; healthcare capacity; how well it abides by public health norms, such as sharing biological samples and reporting outbreaks to relevant authorities; country-specific environmental risks; and political stability. Unsurprisingly, high-income democracies monopolise the top of the table.

Since countries report Covid-19 deaths in different ways, one fair way of comparing outcomes is to compare the number of excess deaths between countries (as measured against a historical baseline determined by mortality rates in previous years). A tracker compiled by *The Economist* takes information from countries that count deaths from all causes and estimates how many excess deaths per 100,000 happened in each of those reporting countries in the period between the first 50 Covid-19 deaths and now.

Figures up to 11 May 2021 showed the US suffered 182 excess deaths per 100,000 people; in the UK, it was 180. They are not the worst performers: countries in the Americas and Eastern Europe fare badly, with Peru (503), Bulgaria (433) and Mexico (354) occupying the top three places on this particular data dashboard. What is staggering is that some countries saw a negative number of excess deaths, suggesting their death rates had gone *down* during the pandemic. They include nations that have drawn global admiration for their Covid-19 responses: New Zealand (–40), Taiwan (–25), Iceland (–14), South Korea (–9) and Singapore (–7). Looking at Scandinavia, I wish the UK had paid more attention to Norway (–19) and Finland (18) than to Sweden (102).

The tracker notes that few countries outside Europe and the Americas release data on excess deaths; in large parts of Asia and Africa, many deaths go unrecorded. There is no data for China, for example. But Johns Hopkins University Coronavirus Resource Center estimates that, as of 30 May 2021, China has had around 103,000 confirmed cases and under 5,000 deaths. The comparable figures for the US are 33 million cases and nearly 600,000 deaths. For the UK, it is close to 4.5 million cases and 128,000 deaths. Even if China, with four times the population of the US, was underreporting its cases by a factor of 20, it would still be doing, per capita, far better than both the US and UK. The pandemic still has a long way to run: one trend to watch is whether the countries thought to have handled the outbreak well, by applying tight border controls and strict in-country measures, are able to vaccinate quickly enough to continue their smooth journey out of the pandemic.

Preparedness metrics simply do not capture how countries responded in real life, says Maria Van Kerkhove, from the Health Emergencies Programme at the WHO, who has become one of the public faces of the pandemic: 'There's a big difference between preparedness readiness and response. The idea that preparedness is something that begins and ends is false. Preparedness and readiness is a constant, and needs to be part of the fabric of society. There's no peacetime anymore. That doesn't mean staying in lockdown or living in fear. But it does mean putting in the investments, so when outbreaks happen countries can act aggressively and comprehensively to minimise the impact. We did not need to be in this level of a global pandemic. It still doesn't need to be this bad.'

The WHO issued a global strategy, basically a plan of public health steps for countries to follow, on 4 February 2020. It was applied, Maria says, by many of the countries that did well: 'There's no rocket science or secret or magic solution. These were tried-and-tested public health actions. If you don't take those actions and if you wait, it gets worse.'

※ ※ ※

Risk registers are no longer enough. We need hard-nosed independent assessments of capabilities, through civil contingency exercises (pandemic war games). These should include a judgement on political and structural capability, which was lacking in the UK through much of this crisis (and throughout, among some ministers). At one stage, politicians focused, with tunnel vision, on getting to 100,000 tests a day without apparently stopping to think why those tests were being done. If tests are being carried out in the wrong place in the wrong way on the wrong people, they can do more harm than good. At that Downing Street meeting with companies selling rapid tests, I saw the same lack of strategic thinking from Boris Johnson. He sat in the middle of the table waving his arms around as he put in offers to buy millions of unproven rapid tests, brushing off the concerns of others in the room who felt, rightly, that test kits needed proper quality control.

The other thing we needed on the first day was a command-and-control structure that ensured action was swift and coherent across government. Instead, the early part of the pandemic was organisational mayhem, with a combination of an absent prime minister, dysfunctional state apparatus and multiple departmental fiefdoms. The lines of responsibility seemed not just blurred but invisible, despite the best efforts of many superb civil servants.

I tried to highlight this by emailing or WhatsApping Number 10 directly, often to Dominic Cummings or Ben Warner. In April 2020, I implored Number 10 to:

move UKG from reactive, announcement drive responses to a strategy! ... I still don't see that central coordination. Still got ministers thinking and acting as if in campaign mode, another announcement, it's all ok ... it needs some grown-ups to set out a 12-month strategy.

Matt Hancock shoulders a responsibility for the PPE shortages and testing fiasco, among other failings, that contributed to the dreadful epidemics in care homes and hospitals. Contrary to his assertions, asymptomatic transmission was understood by mid-February (thanks to the *Diamond Princess*). But the Cabinet Office also failed to provide coordination, with the Cabinet Office minister Michael Gove keeping a noticeably low profile during the pandemic. This was not just a health crisis but one that affected every aspect of society: health, social care, schools, jobs, hospitality, travel, transport, the economy.*

Through that direct line to Number 10, I was also pushing for things to be set up quickly, outside government departments if need be. A crisis on this scale needs talented people working on defined tasks who can make quick decisions unencumbered by bureaucracy, Notably, many of the UK's biggest successes during the pandemic were achieved by teams working outside formal government structures and agencies: the Vaccines Taskforce, led by Kate Bingham; the RECOVERY trial set up in a matter of days by Martin Landray and Peter Horby; COG-UK, initiated quickly by Sharon Peacock beyond PHE, which is keeping tabs on the variants; and the Office for National Statistics infection studies.

Patrick Vallance and Chris Whitty deserve enormous credit for championing and supporting these initiatives. While I thought Chris was a bit slow in January and February to grasp the gravity of the coronavirus outbreak, both have done a remarkable job in helping to steer the country through this crisis under unrelenting pressure, and despite the lack of clarity about how SAGE advice was absorbed into policy making. They have also weathered a barrage of unwarranted personal attacks. Since April 2020, Chris and Patrick have worked fantastically well together, kept SAGE focused and been clear and transparent about what is happening. Angela McLean, the chief scientific adviser at the Ministry of Defence, and Jonathan Van-Tam, England's deputy chief medical officer, have also handled being in the public eye with honesty, professionalism and integrity.

---

* The lessons from the pandemic are summarised well in a report from the Institute for Government, with whom the Wellcome Trust will be working on this topic.

The full story of this historic crisis, particularly the delays that preceded the second lockdown, despite the wealth of data pointing to imminent disaster, demand an immediate public inquiry. This book has tried to shed further light on those delays.* Many of the UK's Covid-19 deaths happened in January, February and March of 2021; they were avoidable. The political decisions made, or not made, in the second half of 2020 were unforgivable.

We must not become numb to the statistic of 127,775 lost lives that introduces this chapter. Each one represents a cherished person with a family, friends, hopes, ambitions and, perhaps, foibles and regrets. These were mothers, fathers, daughters, sons, sisters, brothers, aunts, uncles, grandmothers and grandfathers, neighbours, confidantes and colleagues. These were people. The unique fullness of each life, and the unique horror of its disappearance, cannot be captured in numbers. They must not be written off as collateral damage or a statistic.

Prime minister Boris Johnson has announced that a public inquiry will start in 2022. It is a disgrace it will take that long. There is absolutely no reason, other than political manoeuvring, to wait.† An inquiry into the UK's handling of the Covid-19 pandemic will not be anywhere near as complex as the Chilcot Inquiry into the war in Iraq, which had national security considerations. This is public health. The inquiry could start now, issue an interim report in six months so that we can fix things quickly, and report fully after twelve months. Everyone needs to learn the lessons,

---

* They are also covered in some detail in the book *Failures of State* (HarperCollins, 2021) by the *Sunday Times* journalists Jonathan Calvert and George Arbuthnott.

† Johnson claimed the delay was so that '[We do] not inadvertently divert or distract the people on whom we depend in the heat of our struggle against this disease ... it would not be right to devote the time of people who are looking after us, who are saving lives, to an inquiry.'

scientists included. We only honour the dead by pledging to learn from the mistakes that cost them their lives.

The UK and the world needs to interrogate what happened, because all of us must be ready next time, whenever that next time comes. Protecting lives, and our way of life, is infinitely more important than protecting reputations. There is no natural law governing when the next outbreak will arrive, who it will affect and how catastrophic it will be. A virus could leap across from animals to humans somewhere in the world and begin spreading tomorrow, or later this year, or in 2024. Our urbanised, interconnected world is custom-built for pandemics.

My fears about Africa, which I mentioned so often in my circulars to close colleagues, have not panned out: it has been affected by Covid-19 less than expected. I do not rule out worse to come, though, especially if new, fiercely transmissible variants circulate, the health systems on the continent remain fragile and the vaccine spoils of humanity's war against the virus are not shared equitably.

John Nkengasong, director of the Africa Centers for Disease Control and Prevention, is certainly not complacent: 'This is a war and there are battles before you win. In the first battle, Africa has resisted. But we don't know what the second battle will look like.' He believes the continent's young population, with a median age of 20 years, bore the brunt of infections, providing a buffer or wedge against wider circulation. He is, however, chastened by the devastation in India in early 2021, which came after a relatively modest first wave.

His fear is that the uncertainty around vaccine delivery, and the inability to plan a complex roll-out in advance, may have two serious consequences: that, as the Global North vaccinates, it will demand vaccine certificates to resume trade and travel and therefore worsen inequalities in a world of vaccine haves and have-nots; second, that large amounts of virus will continue circulating among people infected with HIV, brewing monstrous new variants in people who take a long time to clear infections.

John's message to the G7 is clear: redistribute existing vaccine doses and release $50 billion now to get vaccine manufacturing capacity up and running across the world in the next year: 'We have the tools to win this war against the pandemic. First, we must redistribute the vaccines that countries are sitting on. The lack of vaccines is a serious burden for Africa, but if other countries do not share them, it will become a serious moral burden for them.

'Second, in this time of need, we must spend to strengthen capacity. If we cannot be bold and think big during this pandemic and do the equivalent of sending a man to the moon, then I don't think we are taking this pandemic seriously.'

❊ ❊ ❊

I have thought a lot about things I wish I had done differently: discussed travel bans and border controls more extensively much earlier (possibly in January 2020, even though the WHO was advocating against them); argued vigorously for better preparations in February 2020, a wasted month; pushed harder for an earlier lockdown in March 2020, because doing that even one week earlier in the first wave would have saved thousands of lives; learned more from other countries, including China, which would have challenged my prejudices about which infection control measures are acceptable in western democracies; probed harder for evidence that the epidemics in UK hospitals and care homes were under control, rather than taking claims on trust. I wish I had appreciated earlier that some people in Number 10 thought herd immunity, or 'taking it on the chin', was a viable strategy. The idea has no basis in science and absolutely did not come from SAGE. I still do not know where it came from.

I wish I had challenged the lack of testing more robustly and questioned why community testing was being abandoned. Why did one of the leading world economies take so long to have testing in place in hospitals and care homes? Given the Wellcome Trust's work in other areas of the world with devastating outbreaks, and the lessons that I and colleagues have learned about understanding the communities we serve, I wish that ethical considerations had been built into the UK's coronavirus response right from the beginning. Broadly, I think SAGE did well in advocating policy, but perhaps we could have done better in speaking truth to power. Perhaps we could have more clearly communicated the simple mathematics underlying epidemics and warned more trenchantly against optimism bias and confirmation bias. I would like to see future SAGE meetings recorded, not just minuted, and the government's chief scientific and medical advisers given more operational latitude to pull levers to get things done.

There are things we can start doing now: spend money on health, in terms of staff, research and buildings; fix health and other inequalities today, so they are not widened in a crisis tomorrow, as has happened with Covid-19; improve data flows in public health to make timely decisions; coordinate and speed up decision-making across government; unite local and regional authorities with central government (as Australia has done so well); develop a crisis playbook for the Cabinet Office; make supply chains resilient; know when to step outside the usual structures to get things done quickly; be prepared to learn from other countries when it comes to governance and management; practise better crisis messaging.

How did science, as a discipline, acquit itself? The pandemic pushed scientists to their limits, to go as fast and as far as possible. Researchers dropped their usual workloads and joined the international effort. Journals and preprint servers worked hard to build up a critical mass of reliable information and make it freely available at speed. Our knowledge about the virus evolved along with the virus itself, but the uncertainty allowed misinformation and disinformation to flourish. There was great science, which gave us vaccines; there was science that could have been better, like clinical trials, which mostly ended up being patchy and uncoordinated (with the notable exception of RECOVERY and Solidarity* trials); and there was bad science, including speculation, without evidence, that there would be no second Covid-19 wave. Even now, there are still people who sincerely believe that lockdowns do not bring down transmission and that vaccines do more harm than good.

If citizens reject the scientific method, which is at the heart of everything we do and which has given us the means to exit this pandemic, then our future struggles against climate change, water scarcity and diseases will be that much tougher. We need to be more open and engaging about what we do, how the scientific process works, how scientific research and analysis influences policy making and how its benefits can be shared fairly.

In some ways, humanity struck it lucky with Covid-19. The young are relatively protected, perhaps thanks to cross-immunity created through exposure to seasonal coronaviruses. This protective 'memory' fades with age. We have safe and effective vaccines. Future generations of pan-coronavirus vaccines may well shield us from all forms of SARS-like

---

* Solidarity is a WHO-run international clinical trial of treatments for Covid-19.

coronaviruses. In many ways, we can see the light at the end of the tunnel, even if unequal access to vaccines is making the tunnel longer than it needs to be.

But, as Maria Van Kerkhove says: 'This [Covid-19 pandemic] isn't the bad one. It spreads easily but has a relatively low mortality. We could get something much worse.' Imagine if we flipped the age spectrum, so that it was primarily the young, not the old, who were dying in great numbers. Think of how terrifying it would be to see a generation of children and teenagers falling seriously ill; watching hospitals being unable to put young people on ventilators because the health system had imploded; looking on helplessly as the global workforce collapsed. There is a precedent for that scenario. The Spanish flu of 1918, which rippled around the world until 1920, was particularly deadly to infants, young adults and the elderly. We cannot simply hope for the best.

Instead we must plan for the worst. We know what we need to do. In the perpetual battle of the virus versus the people, we have the knowledge and power to bring about a just and fair outcome in favour of *all* the people.

✳ ✳ ✳

10

Omicron Epilogue

11 FEBRUARY 2022

Known global cases: 404,910,528
Global deaths: 5,783,776
Vaccine doses administered: 10,095,615,243
UK cases: 18,220,515; UK deaths: 159,531

ON 25 NOVEMBER 2021, in the middle of the night, an email landed from Tulio de Oliveira, the geneticist at the University of Kwa-Zulu Natal who had been instrumental in identifying the Delta variant. Hospitals in South Africa's Gauteng province were seeing a flood of coronavirus patients, and Tulio, with an overview of viral genome sequences, had spied something disturbing in the data. A new variant looked fitter than Delta, in that it seemed to be successfully infecting – and hospitalising – a population that should have been basking in a high level of immunity acquired from previous waves of infection plus vaccination. It was spreading fast.

Subject: New variant potentially widespread in SA – need activism to stop it and protect the world

Hi Jeremy:
We will release hundreds of genomes by the weekend and this variant is easy to track as it has the S gene dropout, similar to Alpha.

Very concerning as only emerged 2 weeks ago and increasing in prevalence with start of new wave (1000 infections a day). Earlier sample 11 Nov. Discovered this variant on Tuesday and could not go on media because informing government ...

If a new lockdown was needed, Tulio told me, he would demand funding for the poor. He also tipped me off about a paper coming out in the journal *Nature* on World Aids Day, 1 December, highlighting his team's suspicion that immune-suppressed individuals, such as those with cancer or HIV, could be driving the evolution of the pandemic coronavirus. An immune system that cannot eliminate a virus allows an infection to linger, during which time the virus constantly replicates. The longer you play a fruit machine, the higher the chance you will get three cherries in a row. In the same way, the longer an infection lingers in a person unable to shake it off, the more likely it is that a fitter (more transmissible, or more immune-evasive, or more severe, or all three) version of the virus will pop up just by chance.

Omicron, as the new variant was eventually named,* was indeed a fitter version of the SARS-CoV-2 virus, more contagious than even Delta, which it displaced and which had an estimated natural reproduction number of more than 8. Delta, in turn, was much more contagious than the ancestral Wuhan virus that emerged at the end of 2019, which was estimated to have a reproduction number of about 3.

Omicron took transmissibility to staggering heights. Within about thirty days of being named a variant of concern by the World Health Organization, Omicron was in every continent and growing exponentially. The graphs charting the rise in infections were unbelievable: the lines

---

* The Greek letters Nu and Xi were skipped, the former to avoid confusion with 'new' and the latter as Xi is a common surname. WHO has a policy of avoiding 'causing offence to cultural, social, national, regional, professional or ethnic groups'.

were not just exponential but vertical. Omicron, which I did not know of until Tulio's email, kicked Delta off the scene within a month. At the time of writing, in February 2022, it is the dominant variant. But a sub-lineage of Omicron called BA.2 is already displacing it in some areas, highlighting its tremendous capacity for ongoing evolution.

Omicron's origins are unclear, but there are three contending theories. First, it originated in a single chronically ill patient with a lengthy infection; second, it could be the unwelcome product of 'reverse zoonosis', in which the human virus jumped into an animal population, where it gained the bulk of its mutations, and then crossed back into people; or, third, the mutations quietly accumulated as the virus spread from person to person, with this more gradual evolution being missed by sequencing efforts. We do not yet know which is closer to the truth, or whether it originated by some other route.

There are two important factors worth noting about Omicron, which has around fifty mutations, of which more than thirty are on the spike protein. First, it came totally out of left field. Omicron is not a descendant of Delta but instead more similar to the original virus from Wuhan. Its closest known genetic ancestor dates back to mid-2020. It proves something that we already know but that many do not appreciate: evolution is not a linear process and new variants can emerge from anywhere at any time. That should make us wary of chasing variant-specific vaccines.

Second, even though Omicron appears to be less severe than Delta, this is pure chance. This highly plastic virus is only two years old, a short time in the evolution of a virus. Influenza has been with us for millennia. The argument that SARS-CoV-2 will inevitably become less severe is spurious. The way it spreads means that severity is not influencing its evolution ... because the severity comes long after transmission. People often say that a virus doesn't want to kill its host because then it dies; but, if a person is dying a month after transmitting it, severity becomes irrelevant to transmission.

The speed and scale of the Omicron wave calls into question the 100-Days Mission, which is a G7 pandemic preparedness initiative to have vaccines ready to put into arms just 100 days after a pathogen is identified and sequenced. We could achieve close to that now. But, given that Omicron took over the world within a month, I think the real moonshot would be getting from sequencing to global equitable vaccination in that time-frame; or having a vaccine ready for testing in humans within, say, seven days of genomic sequencing, and rolling it out for public health use within a month. There is little glory in patting yourself on the back just for having done something faster than before if it's still slower than the dynamic of the pandemic.

❋ ❋ ❋

By the time Omicron hit, I had stepped down from SAGE. I left the advisory group in September 2021 after having been a member for eighteen months. SAGE has convened longer for the coronavirus pandemic than for any other crisis in its thirteen-year history – by some stretch. When I joined in January 2020, I had the kind of frontline experience of epidemics that many others didn't have, but by autumn 2021 that had changed. Everyone has lived through the pandemic. The challenge to scientific advice no longer needed to come from generalists but from people with deep and detailed expertise, such as John Edmunds on mathematical modelling, or Wendy Barclay, a world-leading virologist researching Covid-19 and flu at Imperial College London.

There were diminishing returns from my continued involvement. The science advice into government was clear and consistent (such as the importance of acting early, lifting restrictions cautiously and in stages, informed by the superb real time data available in the UK) and hasn't really changed. And the expertise inside government has improved. People like Steve Riley,* who made a principled intervention in March 2020 on lockdown timing, are now part of the system. The building blocks of the UK's Covid-19 response are in place: the ONS and REACT studies, genomic surveillance, knowledge of clinical illness; clinical trials; monitoring the NHS; the impact of vaccines; and the studies in care homes and of infection and population immunity.

SAGE was crucial throughout the pandemic but hugely time-consuming for me during a period when Wellcome, a $50 billion organisation, was undergoing substantial reforms and focusing on discovery science and themes such as climate, infections and mental health. I felt I could achieve more by pivoting away from the UK, which was in a pretty good position in terms of science advice, to focus on global sticking points, such as getting vaccines, tests and medicines to the rest of the world. Wellcome has been taking a lead role with the ACT-Accelerator on therapeutics and vaccines, and that needed attention; at one point, I stepped in to become interim chair, and that was a lot of work. It has paid off: the critical goals were to widen access to testing, genomic surveillance, drugs and vaccines. This has happened: in January 2022, COVAX passed the milestone of delivering a billion doses of vaccines.

And, yes, I was fed up with SAGE. Everyone was fed up after eighteen months. It had gone on for a bit too long and had become a bit too big. I talked it over with Patrick Vallance: I felt SAGE needed to slim down, and that my stepping down

---

* Steven Riley, professor of infectious disease dynamics at Imperial College London, joined the UK Health Security Agency as Director General of Data and Analytics.

might give a licence for others. I joked about it later with James Rubin, from King's College London, who felt the same way as I did; he left SAGE just before me and, as we joked, nobody noticed. When it leaked that I had resigned, it made headlines and journalists began ringing everyone I knew (I was on holiday at the time). But it felt a positive step.

Leaving SAGE has given me an extra degree of freedom, particularly in speaking more frankly. When you're locked in the group, you do feel a degree of cabinet responsibility to your peers, although not to the government. I and others stretched it to its limits – to the point that Chris Whitty or Patrick would start meetings by getting up and reminding us of the boundaries on what we could say. They both did it very constructively: as the terms of reference make clear, members of SAGE are free to talk about their own work and to express their views. I and others would never have signed up if we had been gagged.

I haven't spoken to Chris for a while, but I still talk to Patrick regularly, and I haven't stopped contributing to work that feeds into SAGE. I still attend the Thursday-evening phone call in which a group, led by civil servants, pick over data from the ONS, REACT and other surveys.

For what it's worth, I would have opted for Plan B – working from home, mandating masks on public transport and – a week or two earlier than the government did. (It was phased in from 10 December 2021.) But I would not have gone any further than Plan B and certainly would not have advocated futher lockdowns. Omicron looked less severe; the run-up to Christmas is quiet anyway, and workplaces were winding down; schools and colleges were closed; and people were already visibly changing their behaviour in response to the coming surge. Remarkably, the contact patterns over Christmas were similar to those that characterised lockdown, and that just about kept a lid on the situation. Plan B was needed but not more.

In addition to voluntary behaviour change, the UK had lived through the autumn and winter of 2021 with high transmission, certainly higher infection rates than many comparable countries in Europe, which furnished a high level of population immunity (at the cost of continued hospitalisations and deaths; I would rather have achieved it through vaccination). There seemed to be a narrative, a societal acceptance, that 150 to 300 deaths a day was just something that we had to live with. Unless, of course, you or a loved one happened to die from it.

SAGE does what it says on the tin – it's for dealing with emergencies – but I think we need something different now, focused on long-term strategic thinking. I don't think that is happening enough. When you're caught up in the maelstrom of a crisis, it's very difficult to think about what comes next, because, rightly, there's a natural tendency to focus on the here and now of people dying and hospitals overflowing.

But we do need to consider the trajectory of what comes next. We need people who are not knackered and fed up, to have the time and space to actually think, 'OK, this is where we are now, but where do we want to be by next winter, or by the end of the decade? What do we need to accomplish in 2023, 2024 and 2025 that will allow us to get there?'

✳ ✳ ✳

In our haste to return to normal, we have been trying to kid ourselves that this pandemic was a once-in-a-century event, that Covid-19 is becoming endemic – and, well, it wasn't that bad, was it? Endemic does not mean mild; people still die of endemic diseases like tuberculosis and malaria. We are also lulling ourselves into thinking that vaccines on their own will always be able to get us out of it. My biggest concern today is that we underestimate SARS-CoV-2 and then get hit by a new variant (anywhere in the world) that causes severe illness and escapes immunity. Or that we just accept that endemicity means ongoing disruption, sickness and deaths.

So, what are the possible scenarios for how the virus will evolve? Broadly, there are five. In *Scenario 1*, SARS-CoV-2 spontaneously vanishes in the way that SARS-CoV-1 did, after the deadly 2002–4 outbreak (thanks to the fact that infected people only transmitted the disease while symptomatic, which made public health control easier). I would put the chance of SARS-CoV-2 simply disappearing at a whisker above zero. In *Scenario 2*, Covid-19 becomes an endemic disease, with a constant, steady-state turnover of infections, distinct from the spikes and surges that characterise epidemics and pandemics. Global immunity rises, and overall there is less severe disease; there may be flu-like seasonal epidemics, and we might end up vaccinating the vulnerable seasonally, as we do with flu. We might be heading towards this scenario at the moment, but we are definitely not there yet.

In *Scenario 3*, the pandemic virus continues to evolve, producing new variants that lead to new waves of severe illness, hospitalisations and deaths over the coming years, with the virus possibly affecting a wider group of people as immunity wanes, including those not deemed particularly vulnerable.

Scenario 4 also sees continued evolution, through mutations and/or re-combination of two or more variants, producing significantly more dangerous variants that evade immunity to a much greater extent. That would lead to severe disease and deaths, including in younger people and those with prior immunity. This unwelcome possibility could throw up additional risks, such as: immune enhancement, in which a previously infected person suffers more severe disease on reinfection; a new and shifting range of clinical symptoms; or an altered age profile of those affected – for example, an enhanced risk to young people or a more protracted, debilitating long-COVID syndrome.

Scenario 5 is a double whammy: that SARS-CoV-2 continues to circulate, but another, different pathogen emerges or re-emerges nationally, regionally or globally, so that there are two epidemics – perhaps even two pandemics – happening at the same time. The fact that Covid is ongoing doesn't stop another event from happening; the two are completely independent of one another.

There is a very strong public and political desire to focus on the rosier scenarios, like *Scenario 2*. It is the most likely scenario, at least in the UK and similar countries. But the other possibilities are plausible. Scientists and politicians must prepare for them. It would be a tragedy to announce freedom days, pretend it's all over, cross our fingers and pretend the past two years were a bad dream, when there is a chance (even a small non-zero chance) of something awful happening down the line. We would be wrong to allow ourselves to be back in the same position as we were in early 2020.

So what do we need to do? Vaccines – fantastic though they are (and the Omicron onslaught would have been appalling without them) – are not the end of the story. We must not assume the current vaccines are going to be able to do everything for us forever. We need to invest now in next-generation vaccines, including mucosal vaccines, that can offer greater protection and can block transmission. It is transmission, after all, that drives new variants. Second-generation vaccines might be combinations that protect against multiple strains, perhaps folded in with a flu vaccine; third-generation offerings will, hopefully, be pan-coronavirus vaccines that can stop transmission and protect against all past and future variants of SARS-CoV-2.

We have a window of opportunity now. We should spend 2022 studying whether fourth doses of current vaccines are really needed, and how different vaccines can be mixed and matched, given that recent arrivals such as the newly approved Novavax vaccine might offer complementary boosting of the immune system alongside RNA vaccines. I fear that once one country starts to give a fourth dose of RNA vaccine, as Israel and Korea have done, every other country will follow suit whether it's clinically justified or not. That would have a big impact on global supply.

There are other urgent priorities on the science agenda: expanding available therapies and making sure they can be given in combination rather than as monotherapies, to reduce the chances of the virus escaping any single drug; making sure that there is manufacturing capacity for PPE and oxygen; and ensuring sufficient hospital capacity ahead of a possible resurgence later in 2022.

❋ ❋ ❋

The world has seen an unacceptably high number of deaths, in many countries, of people of all ages. In the first quarter of 2022, there will have been 1 million US deaths from Covid-19 – and that's with a high vaccination rate. By comparison, 58,000 Americans died in the Vietnam War, and that changed American foreign policy and politics for decades.

I am fascinated by what's happened to the UK's psyche. We've normalised a level of mortality that would have been totally unthinkable in somewhere like Australia, which has seen fewer than 5,000 deaths so far in total. That attitude is shaped by the context of what's gone before. Given that the UK had more than 1000 deaths a day in early 2021, the current levels of around 200 a day don't appear quite as bad. On top of that, it's human nature to think, 'I've had enough of this virus and I want to move on. I know my individual risk and I can mitigate that by testing before I go and see my grandmother.' You can hear it in the narrative of 'learning to live with the virus'.

Attempts are made to play down people's suffering and there are still some who argue we should allow people to get infected so that natural immunity builds up. The advocates of natural herd immunity never go on to spell out what that means, which is: 'We would accept one in 200 infected people dying, plus long Covid.' The argument that natural infection, rather than vaccination, is the route to salvation underestimates the number of people who wouldn't quite make it. It undercounts, in every community, the number of people living with cancer or HIV; and that babies arrive, with no immunity, every year. It is a callous approach that belongs to the Dark Ages.

It is dangerous to normalise this level of death and illness because it stops us from taking action. People sometimes compare Covid-19 to malaria, which is endemic in many parts of the world. It is not a reassuring comparison: malaria kills around 500,000 a year, mostly under-5s and pregnant women. But, as is implied by the definition of 'endemic', there is a stability to the rates of malaria transmission. That is not yet true of Covid.

Research into malaria also points to the hollowness of a popular argument used to excuse high levels of coronavirus transmission: that people died 'with Covid', not 'of Covid'. This distinction is nonsense. In malaria-endemic regions, many people coming into hospital with, say, a broken leg will have malaria parasites because there's such high community transmission. The fact you've got parasites on board means you're more likely to be anaemic and perhaps a bit underweight – both have a direct impact on how severe that broken leg will prove to be. It is the same with Covid, as intensive care staff already know. Being 'with' Covid affects your recovery from heart attack or stroke. If you have Covid, you cannot start chemotherapy or undergo surgery.

It is not scaremongering to point out that the long-term consequences of this pandemic virus are unknown. We don't understand the causes of long Covid or its implications. We don't know the spectrum of illness that comes under the 'long Covid' umbrella, whether it spans a month of feeling really tired and short of breath to still being breathless six months or a year later. We don't know if sufferers are going to have sub-optimal health five years down the line – and we don't know that there won't be, at some time in the future, a further impact of Covid-19 that we've not yet predicted.

A paper that came out in January 2022 suggests very strongly that infection with the Epstein-Barr virus is linked to multiple sclerosis in later life. Many of the conditions we currently think are either purely genetic or are somehow random in origin might, we find out later, have their origins in infectious diseases or a toxin. Smoking causes lung cancer, as Richard Doll proved; cervical cancer is linked to prior infection with the human papilloma virus.

Who knows whether Covid-19 infection has other nasty surprises in store?

✿ ✿ ✿

On 15 December 2021, on the day that a new UK record was set for the number of coronavirus cases reported in a single 24-hour period (78,000), Boris Johnson announced the chair of the public inquiry into the government's handling of the pandemic. Baroness Heather Hallett, DBE, who earned plaudits for her sensitive handling of the inquiry into the 7 July bombings in London, must now set the terms and scope of this inquiry. But the wheels are grinding slowly and I fear the inquiry is being kicked into the long grass for political reasons. If it takes its usual length of time – two, three or four years – we could be past a general election. We might also, hopefully, be beyond the worst of Covid.

In the meantime, all sides of the political spectrum are already trying to shape the narrative and pre-empt the inquiry's conclusions: anti-vaccination campaigners will claim that vaccine policies were too intrusive, while some on the 'libertarian' right will claim that experts were untrustworthy. I really think we should have had an interim inquiry, so we could stop and figure out what worked, so it could inform the next phase. Any public inquiry must examine, for example, how ministers repeatedly failed to act and then had to take far more draconian action later, including lockdowns, which can and should be avoided.

As it is, I would advocate a time-limited approach so that any inquiry doesn't drag on forever, which risks everybody losing the will to make any reforms because everyone wants to move on. The worst that can happen is that we conclude everything is OK and we bob along in the same way as before. This is the only time – directly after a crisis – when you can really bring about radical change.

The crucial question is: what do we want to get out of the inquiry? We want to learn lessons from before the pandemic, during the acute phase, and the recovery phase. We fundamentally need to understand how we are going to reform the systems and structures within government, whether it's through government decision-making, investment in science, government investment in science and in the public health system, or resilience in our education, supply chains and economic system.

We need to look at the international picture, too, which, thanks to British exceptionalism, we failed to do early on in the pandemic. Why, for example, did Norway, Finland and Denmark do relatively well but Sweden so badly, despite similar demographics? Can we learn from Australia's approach of driving down transmission, vaccinating and then opening up? I think the Australian model is one for other countries to follow. Why was Australia able to make a federal structure work, but not the US? The undermining of the Centers for Disease Control and Prevention (CDC) by the Trump administration made a national approach very hard. The US Covid response has been a disaster, with more than 1 million deaths. What can we learn from Singapore, Vietnam and Taiwan? Or from China's zero-Covid approach and their exit strategy?

The inquiry is also an important moment for those whose voices have been barely heard in the pandemic: bereaved families; frontline workers and healthcare staff; the clinically vulnerable, including those who are shielding; young people; and marginalised communities. Bereaved families have been sidelined and almost regarded as an embarrassment by the UK government. It took until September 2021 for ministers, or Boris Johnson, to meet them. Morale among healthcare workers is unbelievably low and levels of post-traumatic stress disorder frighteningly high. They are people, not robots. There are a lot of people leaving, or taking early retirement, or not taking on additional work, because they cannot face more of the same. A post-Brexit UK can no longer fill those gaps from Europe, so it might need to recruit from low- and middle-income countries. That raises its own ethical questions.

Vulnerable communities have not had a voice, particularly those who have been shielding. They have been sheltering either because they know they must, or because they just don't know if they should. Millions of people in this country have been understandably fearful. It is hard to blame them, given that reported UK cases exceeded 200,000 a day at the height of the Omicron peak.

In terms of young people, the disruption to education will reverberate for years. The UK never prioritised education anywhere near highly enough, as exemplified by pubs being allowed to open while schools were closed. Our number one priority should have been to keep schools and colleges open – for example, by ensuring they were adequately ventilated and with appropriate testing in place. Many schools were built in the nineteenth century to keep the cold air out, rather than to allow fresh air in. We should have vaccinated children more quickly. We give them a flu vaccine to protect them and their families, so why not the Covid-19 vaccine?

Finally, marginalised communities, whether through language or culture, also suffered. Those so-called hard-to-reach communities, particularly ethnic minority communities, have endured the worst health outcomes, and have a lower vaccine uptake. It's not that such communities are anti-vaccine; they are just not sure, and, rather than stigmatising them as hard to reach, we should do more to reach them. The pandemic has widened the cracks in society. We are not all in this together – not in this pandemic, nor those to come.

Globally, we are forgetting and moving on too quickly. We should be reforming the constitutions of financial institutions like the World Bank and IMF, so they can prevent and respond more quickly to events like disease outbreaks, which can destabilise the global economy. The WHO remains chronically underfunded and a pawn in a political system –

although, among transnational institutions, it has come out of the pandemic well. In some ways, it has emerged stronger: it has offered blunt, evidence-based technical guidance, even if many countries did not want to listen; it has corralled the research community; and it has argued strongly for vaccine equity. Tedros has been deservedly re-elected, unopposed, as its director general.

But the geopolitics remains a mess. The G7 and G20 has shown a frustrating inability to be cohesive and act as one. We have assumed accountability rests with nation states and that those nation states will act in the public interest when it comes to international issues. But, in an era of growing nationalism and insularity, where does accountability for cross-border problems actually lie? From where I sit today, I have no confidence the world will handle the next pandemic, or any trans-national issue, including climate change or antibiotic resistance, any better than it has grappled with this pandemic.

Two years after the Covid-19 outbreak was declared a pandemic, we are not yet ready to call an end to it. And we remain terrifyingly unprepared for the next crisis.

❈ ❈ ❈

Notes

CHAPTER 1

p. 7 'Known cases: 4'
ProMED-mail post, 'Undiagnosed Pneumonia – China (Hubei): Request for Information', archive number: 20191230.6864153, 30 December 2019. https://promedmail. org/promed-post/?id=6864153%20 #COVID19

p. 8 'It first appeared in 2002 – and one of its victims, Carlo Urbani, was a good friend of mine.'
www.who.int/csr/sars/urbani/en/

p. 11 '"PROMed" stands for ...'
International Society for Infectious Diseases, 'About ISID'. https://isid. org/about-the-international-society-for-infectious-diseases/

p. 13 'The moderator turned out to be Marjorie Pollack ...'
Debora Mackenzie, COVID-19: The Pandemic That Should Never Have Happened, and How to Stop the Next One, London, Bridge Street Press/Little, Brown, 2020.

p. 14 'The unexplained disease was spreading: 44 patients in Wuhan, up from 27 ...'
www.who.int/csr/don/05-january-2020-pneumonia-of-unkown-cause-china/en/

p. 18 'While Zhang informed Beijing'
Y.-Z. Zhang et al., 'Wuhan Seafood Market Pneumonia Virus Isolate Wuhan-Hu-1, Complete Genome'. National Center for Biotechnology Information (NCBI). www.ncbi.nlm. nih.gov/nuccore/MN908947.1

p. 19 'One of the earliest whistleblowers, ophthalmologist Dr Li Wenliang ...'
Andrew Green, 'Li Wenliang: Obituary', Lancet, 18 January 2020.

p. 19 'Eddie had screenshots of messages on WeChat ...'
Private communication, Eddie Holmes.

p. 21 'SARS is a painful memory in the collective Chinese consciousness...'
Yanzhong Huang, 'The SARS Epidemic and its Aftermath in China: A Political Perspective', in Institute of Medicine (US) Forum on Microbial Threats and S. Knobler et al. (eds), Learning from SARS: Preparing for the Next Disease Outbreak: Workshop Summary. Washington DC, National Academies Press, 2004. www.ncbi.nlm.nih.gov/books/ NBK92479/

p. 25 'Andrew immediately uploaded it to virological.org ...'
Eddie Holmes, 'Novel 2019 Coronavirus Genome'. https:// virological.org/t/novel-2019-coronavirus-genome/319

p. 26 'On 11 January, China CDC sent the genetic sequence privately to WHO...'
World Health Organization, Twitter, 11 January 2020. https://twitter.com/WHO/ status/1216108498188230657

p. 27 'On Saturday 11 January came the first reported death ...'
Andrew Jospeh, 'First Death from the Wuhan Pneumonia Outbreak Reported as Scientists Release

DNA Sequence of Virus. *Stat*, 11 January 2020. www.statnews.com/2020/01/11/first-death-from-wuhan-pneumonia-outbreak-reported-as-scientists-release-dna-sequence-of-virus/

p. 27 'On the day that Zhang's laboratory was shuttered, the WHO released a news update ...'
WHO | Novel Coronavirus – China

p. 28 'The Lancet paper set out, in early January ...'
Jasper Fuk-Woo Chan et al., 'A Familial Cluster of Pneumonia Associated with the 2019 Novel Coronavirus Indicating Person-to-Person Transmission: A Study of a Family Cluster'. Lancet, 24 January 2020. www.thelancet.com/journals/lancet/article/PIIS0140-6736(20)30154-9/fulltext#%20

p. 36 'Look what happened with the SARS-CoV-2 variant B.1.1.7 ...'
Grinch (Global Report Investigating Novel Coronavirus Haplotypes, 'B.1.1.7'. https://cov-lineages.org/global_report_B.1.1.7.html

p. 36 'The UK reported it to the WHO in December ...'
WHO | SARS-CoV-2 Variant – United Kingdom of Great Britain and Northern Ireland

p. 36 'Early scientific papers from China were spelling out its grim clinical consequences ...'
Chaolin Huang et al., 'Clinical Features of Patients Infected with Coronavirus in Wuhan, China'. Lancet, 24 January 2020. www.thelancet.com/journals/lancet/article/PIIS0140-6736(20)30183-5/fulltext

CHAPTER 2

p. 37 'Known cases: 282'
World Health Organization, 'Novel Coronavirus (2019-nCoV): Situation Report – 1, 21 January 2020'. www.who.int/docs/default-source/coronaviruse/situation-reports/20200121-sitrep-1-2019-ncov.pdf

p. 37 'He had changed his plans ...'
World Health Organization, 'WHO Director-General's statement on the advice of the IHR Emergency Committee on Novel Coronavirus'. www.who.int/director-general/speeches/detail/who-director-generals-statement-on-the-advice-of-the-ihr-emergency-committee-on-novel-coronavirus

p. 38 'A PHEIC is defined ...'
World Health OrganIzatIon, 'International Health Regulations Governing the Declaration of a Public Health Emergency of International Concern (PHEIC)'. WHO | IHR Procedures concerning public health emergencies of international concern (PHEIC)

p. 39 'Margaret Chan, Tedros's predecessor, is believed by many ...'
Clare Wenham, 'What We Have Learnt about the World Health Organization from the Ebola Outbreak'. *Philosophical Transactions of the Royal Society B: Biological Sciences*, 372(1721), 26 May 2017. www.ncbi.nlm.nih.gov/pmc/articles/PMC5394645/

p. 39 'The Ebola PHEIC in 2019 ...'
'Ebola Outbreak in the Democratic Republic of the CongoDeclared a Public Health Emergency of International Concern'. www.who.int/news/item/17-07-2019-ebola-outbreak-in-the-democratic-republic-of-the-congo-declared-a-public-health-emergency-of-international-concern

p. 40 'And then came a dramatic update..."
Lily Kuo, 'Coronavirus: Panic and Anger in Wuhan as China Orders City into Lockdown'. *Guardian*. www.theguardian.com/world/2020/jan/23/coronavirus-panic-and-anger-in-wuhan-as-china-orders-city-into-lockdown

p. 42 *'I appeared at a press conference at Davos ...'*
'Press Conference: Coronavirus (COVID-19)/DAVOS 2020'. *YouTube.* www.youtube.com/watch?v=BDQtXzu6z08

p. 43 *'His company had quietly picked up the genetic sequence ...'*
'Moderna Announces First Participant Dosed in NIH-led Phase 1 Study of mRNA Vaccine (mRNA-1273) Against Novel Coronavirus'. *Moderna.* https://investors.modernatx.com/news-releases/news-release-details/moderna-announces-first-participant-dosed-nih-led-phase-1-study

p. 44 *'He was referring to a 2007 study on how 43 US cities ...'*
Howard Markel et al., 'Nonpharmaceutical Interventions Implemented by US Cities During the 1918-1919 Influenza Pandemic'. *JAMA Network.* https://jamanetwork.com/journals/jama/fullarticle/208354

p. 48 *'Moderna was about to tout for more investment ...'*
Drew Singer, 'Moderna Prices Its $1.3 Billion Share Sale to Fund Virus Vaccine'. *Bloomberg.* www.bloomberg.com/news/articles/2020-05-19/moderna-stock-offering-is-said-to-price-at-76-per-share?sref=VCvLK5dI

p. 51 *'Except that this pathogen had surfaced in Wuhan ...'*
David Cyranoski, 'Inside the Chinese Lab Poised to Study World's Most Dangerous Pathogens'. Nature, 542, 23 February 2017, pp. 399–400. www.nature.com/articles/

p. 60 *'Among a bunch of preprints on BioRxiv ...'*
Peng Zhou et al., 'Discovery of a Novel Coronavirus Associated with the Recent Pneumonia Outbreak in Humans and its Potential Bat Origin'. *BioRxiv: The Preprint server for Biiology.* www.nature.com/articles/s41586-020-2012-7

p. 61 *'And then Kristian delivered his denouement ...'*
Kathryn E. Follis, Joanne York and Jack H. Nunberg, 'Furin Cleavage of the SARS Coronavirus Spike Glycoprotein Enhances Cell–Cell Fusion but Does not Affect Virion Entry'. *Virology*, 350(2), 5 July 2006, pp. 358–369.

CHAPTER 3

p. 62 *'Known cases: 7,834'*
World Health Organization, 'WHO Director-General's Statement on IHR Emergency Committee on Novel Coronavirus (2019-nCoV)', 30 January 2020. www.who.int/director-general/speeches/detail/who-director-general-s-statement-on-ihr-emergency-committee-on-novel-coronavirus-(2019-ncov)

p. 62 *'Germany's Patient Zero ...'*
Michelle Martin, 'Man in Germany Contracts Coronavirus in One of First Cases Outside China'. *Reuters*, 28 January 2020. www.reuters.com/article/china-health-germany-idINKBN1ZR04Y

p. 62 *'At last, the Emergency Committee was unanimous ...'*
World Health Organization, 'Statement on the Second Meeting of the International Health Regulations (2005) Emergency Committee Regarding the Outbreak of Novel Coronavirus (2019-nCoV)'. www.who.int/news/item/30-01-2020-statement-on-the-second-meeting-of-the-international-health-regulations-(2005)-emergency-committee-regarding-the-outbreak-of-novel-coronavirus-(2019-ncov)

p. 70 *'On 17 March 2020, in a clear, short paper ...'*
Kristian G. Andersen et al., 'The Proximal Origins of SARS-CoV-2'. *Nature Medicine*, 17 March 2020. www.nature.com/articles/S41591-020-0820-9

p. 74 'There has been intense focus on the work of Shi Zhengli ...'
Jonathan Calvert and George Arbuthnott, *Failures of State: The Inside Story of Britain's Battle with Coronavirus*, London, Mudlark/HarperCollins, 2020.

p. 75 'A joint WHO/China report ...'
World Health Organization, 'WHO-Convened Global Study of Origins of SARS-CoV-2: China Part', 30 March 2021. www.who.int/publications/i/item/who-convened-global-study-of-origins-of-sars-cov-2-china-part

p 76 'One reason why rumours persist ...'
Nidhi Subbaraman, 'Heinous! Coronavirus Researcher Shut Down for Wuhan-Lab Link Slams New Funding Restrictions'. *Nature*, 21 August 2020. www.nature.com/articles/d41586-020-02473-4

p 76 'In May 2021, several scientists including Ralph Baric ...'
Jesse D. Bloom et al., 'Investigate the Origins of COVID-19'. *Science*, 372(6543), 14 May 2021. https://science.sciencemag.org/content/372/6543/694.1

p. 78 'On 5 February 2020, the Diamond Princess ...'
Kenji Mizumoto et al., 'Estimating the Asymptomatic Proportion of Coronavirus Disease 2019 (COVID-19) Cases on Board the *Diamond Princess* Cruise Ship, Yokohama, Japan, 2020'. *Eurosurveillance*, 25(10), 12 March 2020. www.eurosurveillance.org/content/10.2807/1560-7917.ES.2020.25.10.2000180

p. 85 'Researchers would later count more than 1,300 separate occasions ..
Hannah Devlin, 'No "Patient Zero" as Covid-19 Came into UK at Least 1,300 Times'. *Guardian*, 11 June 2020. www.theguardian.com/world/2020/jun/11/british-clampdown-on-non-essential-travel-came-a-week-too-late

CHAPTER 4

p. 87 'Known cases: 80,239'
World Health Organization, 'Coronavirus Disease 2019 (COVID-19): Situation Report – 36', 25 February 2020. www.who.int/docs/default-source/coronaviruse/situation-reports/20200225-sitrep-36-Covid-19.pdf

p. 87 'The Scientific Advisory Group for Emergencies is an ad hoc group of scientist and experts ...'
Institute for Government, 'Scientific Advisory Group on Emergencies (SAGE)'. www.instituteforgovernment.org.uk/explainers/sage

p. 89 'Neil, who had also been involved in the early WHO response, had been quick off the mark ...'
Kate Hodel et al., 'Coronavirus: More Cases and Second Death Reported in China'. *Guardian*, 18 January 2020. www.theguardian.com/world/2020/jan/17/corona-second-death-in-china-after-sars-like-outbreak

p. 90 'The UK, meanwhile, was clocking up its first known cases ...'
Chris Tighe et al., 'First UK Cases of Coronavirus as Pair Treated in a Newcastle Hospital'. *Financial Times*, 31 January 2020. www.ft.com/content/353b0438-441e-11ea-abea-0c7a29cd66fe

p. 98 'A SAGE meeting on 5 March brought news of 115 known cases in the UK
'Coronavirus: UK Moving Towards "Delay" Phase of Virus Plan as Cases Hit 115'. *BBC News*, 5 March 2020. www.bbc.co.uk/news/uk-51749352

p. 99 'SARS-CoV-2 had arrived in Italy with a vengeance.'
Vincent Wood, 'Coronavirus: Italy Planning to Quarantine Entire Lombardy Region, as UK Cases Hit 209 and New York Declares Emergency'. *Independent*, 7 March 2020.

www.independent.co.uk/news/world/
europe/coronavirus-italy-quarantine-
lombardy-milan-venice-outbreak-
latest-draft-decree-a9385011.html

p. 104 'Herd immunity by natural
infection is a possible consequence'
Secunder Kermani, 'Coronavirus:
Whitty and Vallance Faced "Herd
Immunity" Backlash, Emails
Show'. BBC News, 23 September
2020. www.bbc.co.uk/news/uk-
politics-54252272

CHAPTER 5

p. 107 'Known global cases: 113,702'
World Health Organization,
'Coronavirus Disease 2019
(COVID-19): Situation Report – 50',
10 March 2020. www.who.int/
docs/default-source/coronaviruse/
situation-reports/20200310-sitrep-
50-Covid-19.pdf?sfvrsn=55e904fb_2

p. 126 'Jeremy's successor, Mark
Sedwill, seemed to me, absent...'
George Parker et al., 'Inside
Westminster's coronavirus blame
game'. Financial Times, 16 July
2020. www.ft.com/content/
aa53173b-eb39-4055-b112-
0001c1f6de1b

p.128 Cummings's opinions on
controversial scientific issues have
raised eyebrows.
'Dominic Cummings criticised
over 'designer babies' post' www.
theguardian.com/politics/2020/feb/19/
sabisky-row-dominic-cummings-
criticised-over-designer-babies-post

p. 132 'If we needed yet another
compelling reason to act, Report 9
fitted the bill.'
Mark Landler and Stephen Castle,
'Behind the Virus Report that Jarred
the UK and US to Action'. New
York Times, 17 March 2020. www.
nytimes.com/2020/03/17/world/
europe/coronavirus-imperial-college-
johnson.html

p. 134 'Instead, when Boris Johnson
appeared on TV ...'
'Coronavirus: PM Says Everyone
Should Avoid Office, Pubs and
Travelling'. BBC News, 16 March
2020. www.bbc.co.uk/news/uk-
51917562

CHAPTER 6

p. 135 'Known global cases:
167,515'
'Coronavirus Disease 2019
(COVID-19): Situation Report – 56',
16 March 2020. www.who.int/
docs/default-source/coronaviruse/
situation-reports/20200316-sitrep-
56-Covid-19.pdf?sfvrsn=9fda7db2_6

p. 136 'Behavioural fatigue seems to
have been a peripheral idea ...'
Elisabeth Mahase, 'COVID-19:
Was the Decision to Delay the
UK's Lockdown Over Fears of
"Behavioural Fatigue" Based on
Evidence?' British Medical Journal,
7 August 2020. www.bmj.com/
content/370/bmj.m3166

p. 137 'As London was ahead
of other regions in its number of
infections ...'
George Parker et al., 'Inside
Westminster's Coronavirus Blame
Game'. Financial Times, 16 July
2020. www.ft.com/content/
aa53173b-eb39-4055-b112-
0001c1f6de1b

p. 141 'Consumer spending on food
and medicines was rocketing ...'
Helen Pidd, 'UK Supermarkets
Ration Toilet Paper to Prevent
Stockpiling'. Guardian, 8 March
2020. www.theguardian.com/
world/2020/mar/08/coronavirus-
stockpiling-supermarkets-toilet-
paper-hand-gel

p. 143 'On 6 April, the PM was
rushed to intensive care ...'
'Coronavirus: Boris Johnson
Admitted to Hospital over Virus
Symptoms'. BBC News, 6 April

2020. www.bbc.co.uk/news/uk-52177125

p. 145 'It was a grave error.'
Gabriel Pogrund and Hannah Al-Othman, 'Test and Waste: Dido Harding, Boss of £12bn Tracing Scheme, Says it Was Never a Silver Bullet'. *Sunday Times*, 18 October 2020. www.thetimes.co.uk/article/test-and-waste-dido-harding-boss-of-12bn-tracing-scheme-says-it-was-never-a-silver-bullet-s5n66rnjc

p. 146 'A related problem around that time was the NHSX app ...'
Simon Murphy, Dan Sabbagh and Alex Hern, 'Piloted in May, Ditched in June: The Failure of England's Covid-19 App'. *Guardian*, 18 June 2020. www.theguardian.com/world/2020/jun/18/piloted-in-may-ditched-in-june-the-failure-of-englands-Covid-19-app

p. 148 'On 27 March 2020, against lockdown rules, Dominic Cummings'
Stephen Castle and Mark Landle, 'Dominic Cummings Offers a Sorry-not-Sorry for UK Lockdown Breach'. *New York Times*, 25 May 2020. www.nytimes.com/2020/05/25/world/europe/dominic-cummings-boris-johnson-coronavirus.html

p. 149 'On 5 May 2020, it was revealed that Neil had broken lockdown rules.'
Anna Mikhailova et al., 'Exclusive: Government Scientist Neil Ferguson Resigns After Breaking Lockdown Rules to Meet his Married Lover'. *Daily Telegraph*, 5 May 2020. www.telegraph.co.uk/news/2020/05/05/exclusive-government-scientist-neil-ferguson-resigns-breaking/

p. 153 'These were high points amid the gathering gloom, particularly the RECOVERY Trial ...'
James Gallagher, 'Covid: The London Bus Trip that Saved Maybe a Million Lives'. *BBC News*, 25 March 2021. www.bbc.co.uk/news/health-56508369

CHAPTER 7

p. 158 'Global known cases: 24,854,140'
World Health Organization, 'Coronavirus Disease (COVID-19): Weekly Epidemiological Update', 30 August 2020. www.who.int/docs/default-source/coronaviruse/situation-reports/20200831-weekly-epi-update-3.pdf?sfvrsn=d7032a2a_4

p. 160 'In August 2020, Russia approved its home-grown Covid-19 vaccine, Sputnik V ...'
Ewen Callaway, 'Russia Announces Positive COVID-Vaccine Results from Controversial Trial'. *Nature*, 11 November 2020. www.nature.com/articles/d41586-020-03209-0

p. 160 'A cloud, meanwhile, was gathering over the Oxford-AstraZeneca vaccine ...'
'AstraZeneca Pauses Coronavirus Vaccine Trial, Rollout Doubts Dent Shares'. *Reuters*, 15 September 2020. www.reuters.com/article/health-coronavirus-astrazeneca-idUSKBN260187

p. 174 'Whatever happened behind the doors of Number 10 ...'
'Insight Investigation: 48 Hours in September When Ministers and Scientists Split over Covid Lockdown'. *Sunday Times*, 13 December 2020. www.thetimes.co.uk/article/48-hours-in-september-when-ministers-and-scientists-split-over-covid-lockdown-vg5xbpsfx

p. 187 'The UK strategy, such as it was, seemed doomed ...'
Anjana Ahuja, 'The Pandemic's Darkest Hour is Yet to Come'. *Financial Times*, 4 January 2021. www.ft.com/content/0d519265-60ea-483e-87fb-9f7f94037031

CHAPTER 8

p. 189 'Known global cases: 79,231,893'
World Health Organization,

'COVID-19 Weekly Epidemiological Update – 29 December 2020', 29 December 2020. www.who.int/publications/m/item/weekly-epidemiological-update---29-december-2020

p. 199 'Scientists in the UK have been at the forefront of looking for new variants ...'
Sarah Zhang, 'Now We Can See a Virus Mutate as Never Before'. *The Atlantic*, 9 March 2021. www.theatlantic.com/science/archive/2021/03/massive-global-hunt-variants-under-way/618230/

p. 205 'As Tulio explains, there looks be an apparent convergence ...'
Vaughn Cooper, 'The Coronavirus Variants Don't Seem to Be Highly Variable So Far'. *Scientific American*, 24 March 2021. www.scientificamerican.com/article/the-coronavirus-variants-dont-seem-to-be-highly-variable-so-far/

p. 208 'The spectre of vaccine nationalism ...'
Lynsey Chutel and Marc Santora, 'As Virus Variants Spread, "No One is Safe Until Everyone Is Safe"'. *New York Times*, 31 January 2021. www.nytimes.com/2021/01/31/world/africa/coronavirus-south-africa-variant.html

CHAPTER 9

p. 210 'Known global cases: 165,158,285'
World Health Organization, 'Weekly Epidemiological Update on COVID-19: Edition 42', 1 June 2021. www.who.int/publications/m/item/weekly-epidemiological-update-on-Covid-19---1-june-2021

p. 211 'Rather, the deadly black swan could be a radically different flu ...'
Marc-Alain Widdowson, Joseph S. Bresee and Daniel B. Jernigan, 'The Global Threat of Animal Influenza Viruses of Zoonotic Concern: Then and Now'. *Journal of Infectious Diseases*, Supplement 4, 15 September 2017, pp. S493–S498.

p. 212 'Many of the most serious disease outbreaks within living memory ...'
David Quammen, *Spillover: Animal Infections and the Next Human Pandemic*. London, W. W. Norton & Co, 2012.

p. 214 'Everything starts with smarter surveillance.'
'Britain to Work with WHO on "Pandemic Radar" to Track Diseases'. *Reuters*, 20 May 2021. www.reuters.com/world/uk/britain-work-with-who-pandemic-radar-track-diseases-2021-05-20/

p. 216 UNAIDS, 'COVID-19: Make it the Last Pandemic', press statement, 12 May 2021.
www.unaids.org/en/resources/presscentre/pressreleaseandstatementarchive/2021/may/20210512_independent-panel-pandemic-preparedness-response

p. 221 'One of the most striking outcomes of the pandemic ...'
Amy Maxmen and Jeff Tollefson, 'Two Decades of Pandemic War Games Failed to Account for Donald Trump'. *Nature*, 4 August 2020. www.nature.com/articles/d41586-020-02277-6

Glossary

ACT-Accelerator
Access to Covid Tools-Accelerator

asymptomatic
A person is asymptomatic when they are infected with a disease, and can transmit it, but show no symptoms.

avian influenza, bird flu
A type of influenza caused by viruses adapted to birds. There are three types of influenza viruses known as A, B and C. Bird flu outbreaks, such as H5N1 or H7N9, are usually caused by influenza A viruses and have been known to infect humans, as well.

BSI
behavioural and social interventions

BSL
biosafety level

CEPI
Coalition for Epidemic Preparedness Innovations

CFR
'Case fatality rate' (also sometimes called **case fatality ratio**). This is the number of deaths due to a disease divided by the number of confirmed cases, over a set period. So, if 1 out of 50 confirmed Covid cases dies within 28 days, the CFR is 2 per cent. CFR for Covid-19, and other diseases, can change according to the healthcare available.

China CDC
Chinese Center for Disease Control and Prevention

containment
A disease control strategy aimed at preventing community transmission, such as through tracing the contacts of infected people.

coronavirus
A large family of viruses that circulate in animals, including camels and bats. Seven coronaviruses are known to infect humans: four cause mild to moderate disease, such as common colds; and three cause the more severe diseases SARS, MERS and Covid-19. Coronaviruses are named after their crownlike appearance under powerful microscopes; the virus particles are studded with protein 'spikes'.

COVAX
Covid-19 Vaccines Global Access Facility

Covid-19
Covid-19 stands for 'coronavirus disease 2019', the disease caused by SARS-CoV-2.

dexamethasone
A cheap steroid that improves the chances of survival of the sickest Covid-19 patients.

DHSC
Department of Health and Social Care

Ebola
Can refer to the Ebola virus or the disease it causes (Ebola virus disease). The virus, first identified in 1976, is transmitted from animals (such as fruit bats or non-human primates) to people and can spread from person to person through bodily fluids.

elimination
The stamping out of a disease from a geographical region. The 'zero-Covid' approach by New Zealand is an elimination strategy.

endemic
A disease that exists perpetually in a geographical region. For example, dengue fever is endemic in areas where mosquitoes carry the dengue virus.

epidemic
A sudden increase in cases of a disease that is higher than expected for a particular population in a particular area (outbreaks can be regarded as local epidemics)

eradication
The global extinction of a disease through measures such as vaccination. Smallpox is the only human contagious disease so far eradicated.

exponential
As the number of people infected in an epidemic grows, so does the rate at which the epidemic spreads. An exponential curve starts rising slowly but becomes steep very quickly, which is why epidemics seem to suddenly 'take off'.

furin cleavage site
An unusual site on the spike protein of the SARS-CoV-2 virus, thought to underlie the enhanced ability of the virus to infect human cells. Furin is an enzyme (a type of protein) that triggers the cleaving (or splitting) of other proteins to render them active.

FBI
Federal Bureau of Investigation

GAVI
Global Alliance for Vaccines and Immunization

genome
An organism's complete genetic material.

genome sequencing
The process of 'reading' and spelling out an organism's genetic code. SARS-CoV-2 is an RNA virus that is 30,000 'letters' long. In comparison, the human genome, made of DNA, is 3 billion letters long. Genome sequencing can be used to track a virus as it spreads.

herd immunity
Also called **population immunity**, this is acquired in a population when there are enough immune people to stop transmission of a disease. This is usually achieved through vaccination.

herd immunity threshold
The proportion of a population that must be immune to stop a disease spreading – which is higher for more transmissible diseases.

HIV
'Human immunodeficiency virus', which attacks the immune system. It cannot be cured but can be controlled using drugs. Left untreated, it leads to **AIDS** (acquired immunodeficiency syndrome), a life-threatening condition.

IMF
International Monetary Fund

ISARIC
International Severe Acute Respiratory and Emerging Infection Consortium

JBC
Joint Biosecurity Centre

MERS
'Middle East Respiratory Syndrome', a serious illness caused by the Middle East respiratory virus, a coronavirus first identified in 2012 in Saudi Arabia. The virus, carried by bats, has been documented as passing to humans via camels.

mitigation
When transmission of a disease outpaces containment, mitigation can be the next step. In the absence of drugs or vaccines, mitigation uses non-pharmaceutical interventions (such as social distancing and school closures) to slow down an epidemic and reduce its peak, usually to within healthcare limits.

mRNA vaccine
A vaccine containing messenger RNA, consisting of a small stretch of the genetic code of the target virus that the vaccine is designed to protect against. The mRNA is delivered into the body and uses the body's own cells to generate a small piece of the virus. This does not cause disease, but stimulates the immune system to produce antibodies.

mutation
A change in a genetic code. Random mutations occur in RNA viruses like SARS-CoV-2 as they replicate. Many mutations have no effect; others can give the virus a selective advantage, such as higher transmissibility. This is why some mutated forms of the virus (sometimes referred to as variants) become dominant.

NERVTAG
New and Emerging Respiratory Virus Threats Advisory Group

NHS
National Health Service

NIAID
National Institute of Allergy and Infectious Diseases

NIH
National Institutes of Health

Nipah
Can refer to the Nipah virus or the disease it causes (Nipah virus disease). It has been passed from both pigs and bats to humans and was first recorded in Malaysia in 1998. The spectrum of symptoms runs from asymptomatic to fatal encephalitis (brain inflammation).

NPI
non-pharmaceutical interventions

pandemic
A global epidemic, usually affecting large numbers of people on multiple continents.

Pathogen
A microbe that causes disease.
Bacteria, viruses and fungi are
types of pathogen.

pre-symptomatic
The time period between a
person being infected and the
appearance of symptoms. (Those
who never develop symptoms have
asymptomatic infections.) Carriers
of Covid-19 can be contagious in
the pre-symptomatic period.

PHE
Public Health England

PHEIC
Public Health Emergency of
International Concern

ProMED
Program for Monitoring Emerging
Diseases

R
Effective reproduction number
– the number of new infections
generated (on average) by an infectious person in a population where
there are disease control interventions, such as vaccination and/or
social distancing. Controlling an
epidemic usually means bringing
R to below 1, which represents a
shrinking epidemic, whereas an
R above 1 means the epidemic is
spreading.

RECOVERY Trial
Randomised Evaluation of
COVID-19 Therapy Trial

RNA
Ribonucleic acid, a molecule similar
to DNA but simpler, having only a
single strand rather than the double
strand structure of DNA (famously,
a double helix). Rather than DNA,

some viruses are made from RNA,
such as SARS-CoV-2 and Ebola.

SAGE
Scientific Advisory Group for
Emergencies

SARS
SARS stands for 'severe acute
respiratory syndrome', a serious
disease caused by the coronavirus
SARS-CoV-1.

SARS-CoV-1
The coronavirus that causes SARS.
It is closely related to SARS-CoV-2.

SARS-CoV-2
The coronavirus that causes Covid-
19. Previously known as WN-CoV
(or Wuhan coronavirus) and 2019-
nCoV (or novel coronavirus 2019).

spike protein
Sometimes called the **S protein**, it
appears as thorn-like protrusions
on the surface of the SARS-CoV-2
virus. These 'spikes' unpick the
locks of human cells to start the
infection process and hijack the
cell's own replication machinery
so that it begins making new
copies of the virus. The spike
protein is the bit of the virus
recognised by the human immune
system, which is why Covid-19
vaccines generally target it.

suppression
A more extreme form of
mitigation – along the lines of a
'lockdown' – that aims to quash
transmission completely.

variant
a new form of a virus with one
or more mutations. When a
mutated virus behaves substantially
differently from the ancestral

(original) virus, it can come to be regarded as a new strain.

virus

A parasitic infectious agent which cannot reproduce outside a host (scientists debate whether a virus is a 'living' thing). A virus is made up of a genome inside a capsid, or protein shell.

VOC

variant of concern

VOI

variant of interest

VUI

variant under investigation

WEF

World Economic Forum

Wellcome Trust

A global charitable foundation geared to health research, established in 1936 by pharmaceutical tycoon Henry Wellcome. In 2020, it had an endowment of about £29bn, making it the fourth richest charitable foundation in the world. Jeremy Farrar was appointed director in 2013.

WHO

World Health Organization

WIV

Wuhan Institute of Virology

Zika

The mosquito-borne Zika virus causes Zika virus disease, and is named after the Zika forest in Uganda, where it was first identified in monkeys in 1947. Infections were rare until 2007, with Brazil seeing a record outbreak in 2015.

zoonotic: a zoonotic disease (or **zoonosis**) is one that crosses from one species to another.

Dramatis personae

Tedros Adhanom Ghebreyesus

Director general of the World Health Organization (2017–), whose Emergency Committee declared the new coronavirus emerging in China to be a PHEIC (Public Health Emergency of International Concern) on 30 January 2020. This reminded countries that they had to act under the International Health Regulations, including notifying the WHO of cases. Tedros was a key influence in setting up the ACT-Accelerator and has been a strong advocate of global equitable access to all the tools needed to end the pandemic.

Kristian Andersen

Born in Denmark, and with a PhD from Cambridge, England, Andersen is an immunology professor at the Scripps Research Institute in California. He first raised questions about the way the SARS-CoV-2 virus seems 'designed' to infect human cells and co-authored the key paper 'The proximal origin of SARS-CoV-2', which concluded that the virus had most likely arisen naturally.

Stéphane Bancel

French billionaire CEO and part-owner of US biotech company Moderna, Bancel negotiated CEPI funding to begin work on a novel mRNA-based Covid-19 vaccine shortly after the genetic sequence of the virus was released.

Kate Bingham

British venture capitalist appointed in May 2020 to lead the UK's Vaccine Taskforce, which was notably successful in vaccine procurement, purchasing 367 million doses of seven different vaccines even before clinical trials had confirmed their efficacy.

Brown, Gordon

UK Prime Minister (2007–10) who won international praise for his handling of the 2008 financial crisis. Campaigning today against health and vaccine inequality, he has argued for increased contributions to COVAX by rich countries and an enhanced public health focus for international funding organisations including the World Bank.

Bin Cao

A physician and Vice President and Director of Respiratory and Critical Care Medicine at the China, Japan Friendship Hospital in Beijing, he was involved in setting up studies of the newly-emerged disease in Wuhan and later the early vaccine trials in China. He contributed two important Lancet papers on the disease characteristics.

Chen Zhu

Starting as one of Mao's 'barefoot doctors' in rural China, Chen served as China's Minister of Health between 2007 and 2013. A professor at the School of Medicine of Shanghai Jiao Tong University, he has been active in promoting scientific collaboration between China and the rest of the world.

Christiane Dolecek

Austrian-born professor in tropical diseases at Oxford University whose clinical research focuses on antimicrobial drug resistance. She has been married to Jeremy Farrar since 1998 and in 2011 they together established the Farrar Foundation to support young people in Vietnam and Nepal in education, health, science and recreational activities

Francis Collins

A physician, geneticist and expert on disease genetics, Collins headed the Human Genome Project before becoming director of the US National Institutes of Health. He founded the BioLogos Foundation, which promotes the view that belief in Christianity can be reconciled with acceptance of evolution and science. He was involved in early discussions about the origins of SARS-CoV-2.

Tim Cook

Consultant and professor in anaesthesia and intensive care medicine at the Royal United Hospitals in Bath. A long-time friend of Jeremy Farrar, who confided in him his suspicions of the origins of the virus.

Dominic Cummings

Political strategist who was special adviser to Michael Gove, then became Director of Vote Leave and chief adviser to Boris Johnson on the latter's appointment as PM in 2019. His reputation was damaged by travelling to Durham in March 2020 despite having Covid-19 symptoms, in violation of lockdown restrictions. Cummings left Downing Street in November 2020, since when he has openly criticised both Johnson's leadership and UK government responsse to Covid-19.

Richard Danzig

A former Secretary of the US Navy under Bill Clinton and adviser to Barack Obama, Danzig saw that the main obstacle to ending the pandemic would be the supply of vaccines, and proposed a Manhattan Project for vaccines, elements of which survived in Operation Warp Speed, the US project to deliver 300 million doses of vaccines by January 2021.

Peter Daszak

A British zoologist, consultant and expert on zoonoses. He is a president of the non-profit research organisation, the EcoHealth Alliance, which had funded research at the Wuhan Institute of Virology and was a member of the WHO delegation to China.

Tulio de Oliveira

A member of the WHO Virus Evolution Working Group on SARS-CoV-2, Tulio detected what is now called the Beta variant in South Africa and warned colleagues that that the virus appeared to be changing significantly, developing mutations that might allow variants to resist neutralising antibodies. Alarmed by ongoing evolution of the virus, he believes the best solution is to try to eliminate transmission

Ian Diamond

Professor Ian Diamond is the UK's National Statistician, Permanent Secretary at the Office for National Statistics, Chief Executive of the UK Statistics Authority and an executive member of its Board. ONS's infection survey employed random sampling of the UK population.

Christian Drosten

Professor Christian Drosten directs the Institute of Virology at the Charité Hospital in Berlin. He was one of the international group who initially discussed the idea that Covid-19 could be a laboratory-engineered virus.

John Edmunds

A professor in the Faculty of Epidemiology and Population Health at the London School of Hygiene & Tropical Medicine,

Edmunds serves on SAGE and SPI-M. His modelling has been critical to informing the UK's coronavirus response.

Michael Farzan

Professor Farzan is Chair of the Department of Immunology and Microbiology at the Scripps Research Institute's Florida Campus. He made important discoveries about how SARS-CoV-1 binds to human cells and contributed to early discussions about the origins of SARS-CoV-2.

Anthony Fauci

An immunologist who made important advances in patient management in infectious diseases, Fauci is director of the US National Institute of Allergy and Infectious Diseases. A key member of Trump's Coronavirus Task Force, he is now chief medical adviser to President Biden. Involved in early discussions about the origins of SARS-CoV-2.

Mike Ferguson

Professor of Life Sciences at the University of Dundee, expert on protozoan parasites and, since 2018, deputy chair of the Wellcome Trust. Involved in early discussions about the origins of SARS-CoV-2.

Neil Ferguson

British epidemiologist and professor of mathematical biology and immunological modelling at Imperial College in London. He served on SAGE until May 2020, when he resigned after violating lockdown rules. His modelling has been critical to informing the UK coronavirus response.

Ronald Fouchier
Professor of molecular virology at Erasmus Medical Centre in Rotterdam in the Netherlands, who has conducted gain-of-function research. His work showed that that a few mutations can make H5N1 bird flu transmissible through the air between ferrets. Involved in early discussions about the origins of SARS-CoV-2.

George F Gao (Gao Fu)
Chinese virologist and immunologist, who studied at Oxford and Harvard before returning to China in 2004. He became Dean of the Savaid Medical School of the University of Chinese Academy of Sciences in 2015 and Director of the Chinese Centre for Disease Control and Prevention from 2017.

Robert (Bob) Garry
Based at Tulane University in Louisiana, he was involved in early discussions about the origins of SARS-CoV-2. With Kristian Andersen, Andrew Rambaut, Ian Lipkin and Eddie Holmes, he co-authored a paper 'The Proximal origin of SARS-CoV-2', published in March 2020.

Michael Gove
A former journalist, MP for Surrey Heath since 2005 and Minister for the Cabinet Office since 2020. In this book he is remarkable largely for his absence. The Cabinet Office should have provided a coordinating function but Gove kept a low profile during the pandemic.

Timothy Gowers
British mathematician and Fields medallist, he was one of three outside scientists whose views Dominic Cummings sought during the Covid-19 crisis. He told Cummings in a series of emails that the best strategy was to go in hard and early on interventions like lockdowns, because of exponential growth in case numbers.

Sunetra Gupta
Professor of theoretical epidemiology at Oxford, Gupta was one of three academics responsible for the Great Barrington Declaration, which proposed allowing the virus to sweep through the population quickly so that herd immunity could build up, while the vulnerable were shielded. Her claim that half the UK population had already been infected and therefore acquired immunity was contradicted by antibody evidence.

David Halpern
Head of the UK government's Behavioural Insights team (often called the 'nudge unit'), he gave the first interview that mentioned herd immunity.

Matt Hancock
MP for West Suffolk since 2010 and Secretary of State for Health and Social Care since 2018. On 19 March 2020, he introduced the Coronavirus Bill, giving the police sweeping powers,

to the UK Parliament. On 27 March 2020, Hancock and Boris Johnson revealed they had tested positive for coronavirus; Hancock suffered mild symptoms. Dominic Cummings has, notoriously, been scathing about Hancock's abilities.

Baroness Diana 'Dido' Harding

The former chair of NHS Improvement, Harding was appointed to chair NHS Test and Trace following the centralisation of testing on 7 May 2020. Despite its lacklustre performance, she was later appointed head of Public Health England's replacement, the National Institute for Health Protection.

Jenny Harries

A deputy chief medical officer for England. Harries said publicly that the UK did not need to follow the WHO's advice (that countries should 'test, test, test') because it did not apply to high-income countries. In 2021, she was appointed chief executive of the UK Health Security Agency.

Demis Hassabis

A former child chess prodigy, neuroscientist, games designer and entrepreneur, and co-founder of artificial intelligence start-up DeepMind. Hassabis attended the SAGE meeting on 18 March 2020, where he expressed alarm at the way the epidemic was unfolding.

Richard Hatchett

CEO of CEPI (the Coalition for Epidemic Preparedness Innovations) and a former White House adviser (during the H1N1 outbreak of 2009). He concluded a funding agreement with Stéphane Bancel of Moderna in January 2020 and shortly afterward began to include Jeremy Farrar in US emails on the emerging threat and on vaccine development.

Eddie Holmes

British-born evolutionary biologist, virologist and professor at the University of Sydney. Since 2012, Holmes has worked closely with Professor Zhang at Fudan University, Shanghai, on finding and identifying new animal viruses. When China seemed reluctant to publish the Covid-19 genome sequence, he released it on virological.org. He co-authored the Nature Medicine paper 'The Proximal Origin of SARS-CoV-2'.

Peter Horby

Epidemiologist who worked for the WHO in Hanoi and is now an Oxford University scientist. He chaired NERVTAG (New and Emerging Respiratory Virus Threats Advisory Group) meetings, and with Martin Landray pioneered lifesaving studies in the RECOVERY (Randomised Evaluation of Covid-19 Therapies) drug therapy trial. He was also a director of ISARIC (the International Severe and Acute Respiratory and Emerging Infection Consortium) which aims to get clinical trials running quickly.

Boris Johnson

Educated at Eton and Oxford, Johnson is a journalist and

columnist (*Daily Telegraph*, *Spectator*) turned politician. He has been an MP (2001–08, 2015–), Mayor of London (2008–16), and was prominent in the Vote Leave campaign that led to Brexit. He became prime minister in July 2019, so led the country throughout the Covid-19 pandemic. He was himself hospitalised with Covid-19 in April 2020. His handling of the pandemic, particularly the timing of key decisions, has been repeatedly challenged.

Maria Van Kerkhove
Leads the WHO's Health Emergencies Programme and was in contact with Jeremy Farrar as news of human-to-human transmission of Covid-19 emerged. She has expressed surprise at the 'idiosyncratic' British approach to the pandemic and urges constant preparedness as part of the fabric of society.

Marion Koopmans
A virologist at Erasmus University in the Netherlands, Koopmans is a member of the Covid-19 Emergency Committee and has played a key role in researching the origins of the virus. She was part of the WHO team sent to China to investigate. She researches the connection between disease and ecology (how people and animals relate to their environment) and is concerned about other unknown animal viruses.

Martin Landray
An epidemiologist, professor of medicine and member of

NERVTAG, chaired by Peter Horby, with whom he pioneered lifesaving studies into potential treatments for Covid-19 in the RECOVERY (Randomised Evaluation of Covid-19 Therapies) trial.

Eliza Manningham-Buller
Chair of the Wellcome Trust (October 2015 to April 2021) and former director general of the British intelligence service MI5. She advised the author on security issues and concerns about the effectiveness of participation in SAGE. She was succeeded as chair of Wellcome by Julia Gillard, former prime minister of Australia.

Carter Mecher
A doctor and former public health adviser in the US Department of Veteran Affairs, Mecher worked on pandemic preparedness under George W Bush. He produced a comparison of SARS, MERS and Covid-19 derived from case numbers pulled from ProMED-mail and various blogs suggesting the new coronavirus was taking off faster than SARS and that some asymptomatic transmission should be assumed. He proposed 'targeted layered containment'.

John Nkengasong
Cameroon virologist and director of the Africa Centres for Disease Control and Prevention. He sees no reason for complacency about early low levels of infection in Africa, believing the continent's young population bore the brunt of infections and provided a buffer against wider circulation. He is

concerned about future vaccine delivery and roll-out and also that continuing transmission may encourage new variants.

Andrew Parker

Head of the UK intelligence service MI5 after Eliza Manningham-Buller, and met Jeremy Farrar when Wellcome was working on combating Ebola in North Kivu. Wellcome see parallels in understanding security threats and epidemic disease – how to spot the signal among the noise.

Sharon Peacock

Professor of microbiology at Cambridge University, an expert in the genome sequencing of pathogens and an adviser on SAGE. On a two-year secondment to Public Health England, she was director of the National Infection Service and later Director of Science. She set up COG-UK, the Covid-19 Genomics UK Consortium, which has sequenced coronavirus samples in the UK from April 2020. She is concerned about variants posing a risk to vaccine efficiency.

Andrew Rambaut

Professor of Molecular Evolution at the University of Edinburgh, Rambaut runs an open-source website, virological.org, collating information including genome sequences on viruses of interest. In January 2020, he published the coronavirus genome supplied by Eddie Holmes. He countered concerns over the suspicious furin cleavage site by suggesting the virus had acquired it in an

intermediate host species before jumping into humans. He was involved in early discussions about the origins of SARS-CoV-2 and co-author of the paper 'The Proximal origin of SARS-CoV-2' in March 2020.

Steven Riley

A colleague of Neil Ferguson's at Imperial College London and a member of the SPI-M group of modellers, Riley described the Chinese decision to lock down Wuhan as 'the only thing that gave the rest of the world a chance'. In raising the prospect of a China-style lockdown on the basis of the precautionary principle in a note to SPI-M on 10 March, he urged a change of strategy from mitigation to suppression.

Patrick Vallance

Trained as a doctor, Vallance was a clinical researcher at University College London before heading research and development at GlaxoSmithKline. Since 2018, he has been the UK government's chief scientific adviser and ex officio chair of SAGE. He has been praised for his loyal support for other SAGE members and enthusiasm for initiatives like COG-UK.

Jonathan Van-Tam

An expert on respiratory viruses, Van-Tam is (with Jenny Harries) deputy chief medical officer for England. He commented on Cummings's Durham excursion that the rules applied to everyone: public adherence might depend on this principle.

Ben Warner

A data scientist with a doctorate from University College London, Warner worked with Cummings at Vote Leave. He attended SAGE meetings as a Number 10 observer and raised early concerns about the UK's coronavirus response.

Chris Whitty

The UK government's chief medical adviser, Whitty trained in infectious diseases and did a period of study in Vietnam. On SAGE, he initially favoured a cautious approach, but later became convinced that the scenarios that had been modelled would happen. He and Patrick Vallance kept SAGE focused under unrelenting pressure and weathered many personal attacks.

Yong-Zhen Zhang

A professor at Fudan University, Shanghai, and expert in animal viruses, Zhang obtained a sample of the Wuhan virus on 3 January 2020 and had sequenced its genome by 5 January. In close contact with Eddie Holmes, he informed the Chinese Ministry of Health the same day but was prevented from releasing information. He and Holmes released the genome sequence on 10 January 2020 on virological.org.

Acknowledgements

The authors would like to thank Eliza Manningham-Buller for proposing that Jeremy write a book, and Andrew Franklin of Profile Books for bringing us (JF and AA) together to work on this urgent and important project. Huge thanks to Mark Ellingham, our editor, who has steered us calmly from uncertain start to blistering finish. We would also like to thank the following individuals at Profile: Nikky Twyman for proofreading and endnotes; Bill Johncocks for assembling the index and dramatis personae and graciously accommodating last-minute changes; Jack Smyth and Peter Dyer for the spectacular cover design; Henry Iles for text design; Cecily Engle for a careful reading of the manuscript; and Ruth Killick for an expert publicity campaign.

Beyond Profile, we would like to thank our superb specialist editor and fact-checker Mun-Keat Looi, who saved many a blush; Peter Horby, Angela Saini and Eliza Manningham-Buller, who read and commented on earlier drafts of the book. Any mistakes that remain are ours alone.

This book was only possible because of the help, guidance and, on some occasions, the private communications shared by the individuals featured in *Spike*. We have been humbled by their willingness to give up their time to be interviewed, dig out papers and data, explain complex concepts, provide context and, in some cases, correct mistaken assumptions. We are immeasurably grateful to all interviewees and sources, named and unnamed, for their cooperation, trust and support. We earnestly hope that we have not let you down.

We dedicate this book to the healthcare workers, essential workers and scientists across the world who have worked tirelessly in traumatic circumstances to start to bring the Covid-19 pandemic under control. Too many have paid the ultimate price.

From Jeremy
Anj, thank you. It has been amazing working with you. A rollercoaster ride for sure, your wisdom, challenge, and clarity of purpose have been inspirational. I look forward to that dinner and glass of wine.

Heartfelt appreciation to all my colleagues at Wellcome, whose professionalism and dedication to all aspects of our mission and through such uncertain and challenging times has been simply staggering.

Huge respect and enormous thanks to scientists in the UK and around the world who developed and shared the knowledge and now the tools needed to exit from this phase of the pandemic. Scientists have provided the exit strategy, it is now up to politicians to make sure that science is available to everyone, everywhere.

I would like to pay tribute to the extraordinary work of all the members of the Scientific Advisory Group for Emergencies (SAGE), led by Patrick Vallance and Chris Whitty and to so many civil servants across government who worked tirelessly, often unrecognised, under-appreciated and under unrelenting pressure; and to all the partners of the ACT-A, hosted by the World Health Organization, who came together to try and ensure equitable global access to all the tools needed to end the pandemic.

Love to Christiane, our children, our wider families and close friends whose constant support has been so important during some very dark moments as well as during long weekends of joy on the West Coast of Scotland. Thank you to Steeple Aston Cricket Club for pure escapism on occasional Sunday afternoons.

From Anjana
Jeremy, it has been a pleasure and a privilege to work with you on *Spike*. This is a brave and important book and I am proud to be associated with it. Despite the gravity of the subject matter, we managed moments of humour along the way.

Thank you to my agent, Peter Tallack, at the Science Factory for taking on one last coronavirus book!

I would like to thank my colleagues at the *Financial Times* for trusting me on the 'mystery pneumonia' in early January 2020 and for supporting me thereafter to deliver seemingly endless Covid-19 coverage: Brooke Masters (and the lovely team on the Opinion and Analysis desk); Clive Cookson; Donato Paolo Mancini; Alec Russell; and Alice Fishburn. Thanks also to the FT for granting book leave.

Heart-shaped thanks to Tom, Rosa and Seth for putting up with the piles of books and papers, constant Zooming and my chaotic working schedule. The past 17 months have been surreal but there is no-one else I would rather have shared them with. Dearest Rosa and Seth: young people have suffered so much in the pandemic and I am in awe of your resilience.

Mum, thank you for everything. Dad, I miss you. I would have loved to argue about *Spike* with you.

Index

Note: The suffix 'n' indicates a footnote. Where colleagues and friends of the author, after first being introduced in full, are referred to by their given names alone, these have sometimes been provided as duplicate entries or cross-references: thus 'Andrew (Rambaut) see Rambaut'.